Feeding your baby is a very important experience for both of you during the first year of his or her life. But whatever you're offering – breast, bottle, cup, spoon or plate – feeding your baby can be, and often is, a worrying experience with many basic questions unanswered: how do you do it? what food do you give? how much? when? . . .

The A–Z of Feeding in the First Year sets out to answer all the questions that arise during this crucial period. Over 300 entries cover topics from A to Z explaining, defining and describing every aspect of feeding a new baby and the changeover from milk-only to family meals: breast and bottle feeding . . . food intolerance . . . kitchen equipment . . . vegetarianism . . . weight-gain . . . weaning . . . working and breastfeeding. The book includes illustrations and a clearly laid out recipe section for simple, nutritious and tasty dishes for baby and the rest of the family as well.

Many people have problems with breastfeeding that are the result of poor and out-of-date advice; many women prefer not to breastfeed at all; many parents have little time to prepare special meals for their babies. Heather Welford writes for every one of these new parents, offering sound information and sensible advice, with sympathy and humour.

Heather Welford is a writer and journalist in the areas of childcare, family life, health and relationships. She is the Family Editor and 'agony aunt' of *Parents* magazine and has previously published *The Illustrated Dictionary of Pregnancy and Birth* and *Toilet Training and Bedwetting*, and she was a contributing author of *The Mothercare Manual*. She is also a National Childbirth Trust breastfeeding counsellor, and lives in Newcastle-upon-Tyne with her husband and three young children.

Also by Heather Welford
The Illustrated Dictionary of Pregnancy and Birth
(Allen & Unwin, 1986; Unwin Paperbacks, 1987)
Toilet Training and Bedwetting
(Thorsons, 1987)

THE A-Z OF
FEEDING
IN THE
FIRST YEAR

Heather Welford

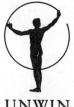

UNWIN
PAPERBACKS

LONDON SYDNEY WELLINGTON

First published in Great Britain by Unwin ® Paperbacks, an imprint of Unwin Hyman Limited, in 1988.

Unwin Hyman Limited
15–17 Broadwick Street
London W1V 1FP

Allen & Unwin Australia Pty Ltd
8 Napier Street, North Sydney, NSW 2060, Australia

Allen & Unwin New Zealand Pty Ltd with the Port Nicholson Press
60 Cambridge Terrace, Wellington, New Zealand

British Library Cataloguing in Publication Data

Welford, Heather, 1952–
  The A–Z of feeding babies
1. Babies. Feeding
I. Title
649.3
ISBN 0–04–440251–1

Printed in Great Britain by Cox & Wyman Ltd, Reading

CONTENTS

INTRODUCTION

The way you feed a new baby and make the change-over from milk-only to family meals isn't a precise science. No one, and no book, can tell you exactly how to do it. There's plenty of room for you to make your own decisions, based on what *you* feel suits you and your baby, without it meaning that you've made a mistake. However, it's helpful to have guidelines around, and some sound information – and that's what I hope this book will give you.

You'll adapt some of the guidelines, you'll use some of the information to help answer queries and solve problems, and above all I hope you'll be helped to enjoy this aspect of your baby's care. Feeding your baby – especially in the early months – is something you do several times a day, and it's an experience you share with him or her whether you're offering breast, bottle, cup, spoon or plate. Too many worries and anxieties can really spoil the pleasure and joy of being a mother.

Because breastfeeding is the best way to feed young babies, I feel it's a great shame more women don't choose to do it, and that many who do give up before they plan to. As recently as four or five years ago, it seemed as though it was only a matter of time before the majority of babies would be exclusively breastfed for the first few months after birth. The trend seemed set fair. But it's become clear, that UK breastfeeding rates have ceased to rise, and there may even have been a significant decline. Perhaps this book will go some way towards providing helpful information about breastfeeding and its problems, so you don't have to rely on poor and outdated advice if you have a problem.

At the same time as accepting the fact that breast milk is superior to anything else we can offer newborns, it's important, I feel, for writers and journalists like myself to acknowledge the right of every mother to choose for herself how to feed, and when and if to make a change to the bottle. Some mothers do make that decision on the basis of what they feel and know is right for them – and of course that needs no justification. It does perturb me, though, that poor information and lack of practical help and support from health professionals, family and friends may mean that the choice is not a totally free one.

Introduction

Weaning – moving on to solids – does worry parents. However, it needn't! In fact, weaning a baby can be an excellent time for the rest of the family to begin eating better. Food intolerance is a topic that's much discussed, and we may have more definite conclusions about its causes and the way to cope with it in a few more years. For the moment, exclusive breastfeeding, followed by gradual weaning, seems the best way of helping your baby avoid developing some form of allergy or intolerance. You'll find more details, of course, in the text.

Babies, in line with real life, are sometimes 'she' and sometimes 'he' in the text.

HEATHER WELFORD

ACKNOWLEDGEMENTS

My three children gave me the practical experience I needed to write this book, so they deserve a 'thank you' at least. The many readers of *Parents* who have written to the 'help' pages I have edited for some ten years now, have shown me what other parents need to know as well.

As regards the text itself, I am grateful to Elisabeth Morse, nutritionist and author. She helped me immeasurably by pointing out woolly thinking, correcting errors and bringing her professional and academic background to bear on my work. The book is a great deal better for her involvement, though of course any errors remaining are my own.

Gillian Clouston and Pat Ford, both home economics teachers, did an excellent job in testing and re-writing the recipes – my thanks to them for this, and to their own babies for eating the results! Both Gillian and Pat contributed some of the recipes themselves. Nicola Dodd, mother of twins, devised several of the recipes as well – again, my thanks.

I also need to thank the mothers I have counselled through my work as a breastfeeding counsellor with the National Childbirth Trust and my many colleagues and friends in NCT. Their experiences have helped me increase my knowledge about breastfeeding, in its social as well as nutritional aspects. However, NCT has had nothing to do with the text, and the book has been written in my professional capacity as a writer only.

Finally, I need to thank my friend and childminder Dorothy Haywood, who looks after my youngest child with love and care while I work. Thanks, too, to my husband Derek Neil, for showing love, tolerance and encouragement throughout this project.

LIST OF ENTRIES

The format of the book is designed to make it easy to dip in as and when you need to look up a specific topic. This does mean that some information is repeated from time to time under different headings – though more often, you will find cross-references in capitals, within or following each entry, to enable you to find out more details if you need them.

Entries with an asterisk (*) after the heading have relevant recipes (see Recipes, page 214).

A

OXYTOCIN

P

PAEDIATRICIAN
  see Help and advice
PARSNIPS*
PARTY FOODS*
PASTA*
PASTRY
PÂTÉ
PEACHES AND NECTARINES*
PEANUT BUTTER
PEANUTS see Nuts
PEAS*
PEPPERS
PERIODS see Menstruation
PINEAPPLE
PKU (Phenylketonuria)
PLATES
PLUMS AND PRUNES*
PORRIDGE
POSITION AT BREAST
POTATO*
POWDERED MILK
PREMATURE BABY
  see Pre-term baby
PRESSURE COOKER
  see Equipment
PRE-TERM BABY
PROLACTIN
PROTEIN
PRUNES see Plums and
  prunes
PUDDINGS see Desserts
PULSES see Beans and
  pulses
PURÉES
PYLORIC STENOSIS

R

RAISINS AND SULTANAS
RASPBERRIES see Berries
REHEATING FOOD
  see Left-overs
RELACTATION
RHUBARB
RICE*
ROOTING REFLEX
ROUTINES
RUSKS*

S

SALADS*
SALT
SANDWICHES*
SCHEDULED FEEDING
SEASONING
SEEDS*
SEMI-SKIMMED MILK
  see Cow's milk
SEX AND BREASTFEEDING
SHARON FRUIT
SICKNESS see Illness; Vomiting
'SICKY' BABY
SKIMMED MILK see Cow's milk
SLEEPING see Colic; Crying;
  Night feeds
SLEEPY BABY
SMOKING
SNACKS*
SOCIETY AND BREASTFEEDING
SODIUM see Salt
SOLIDS
SORE NIPPLES see Nipples
SOUP*
SOYA MILK

The A–Z OF FEEDING
IN THE FIRST YEAR

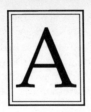

ADDITIVES AND COLOURINGS

In relation to food, an additive is generally used to define anything put in a foodstuff at the manufacturing or processing stage. It doesn't necessarily mean something artificial or grown in a laboratory – SUGAR and SALT, for example, are widely-used additives, and present in many processed foods to change the taste, and also to act as preservatives. In fact, these are the two main reasons why additives are used – to alter the taste of food, and to prevent it going 'off'. They may also be included to alter the appearance of a food, as colourings do, although they are not nutritionally necessary.

Some widely-used additives are associated with ALLERGY and FOOD INTOLERANCE in a few susceptible people. Babies are better off with foods without artificial additives, although that's difficult to prove scientifically. Certainly, no one could possibly do a study with two groups of babies, with one group on foods with lots of additives in them and one on foods with none. But common sense at least tells us that new digestive systems are better off with food that is as close as possible to its natural state. They're better off without added sugar and salt, too, of course. And some natural foods without additives can be damaging to babies if they're given too soon, or given to babies who are intolerant to certain foods. On packaged goods, many additives are listed as 'E' numbers. This is an EEC regulation which allows goods to move within the Common Market without problems. Reading a book like Maurice Hanssen's *E for Additives* explains what each number actually is, and what the known or possible side-effects are in susceptible people.

Artificial colourings have been implicated in cases of food intolerance as well. Tartrazine, the orange colouring in many foods is associated with behavioural disturbances, for example

HYPERACTIVITY. Children who are intolerant to certain foods can react to many different colours, but it's not hard to avoid them if you know that they're not worth the potential problems. If your child needs medication for instance, ask for medicines without added colour. Many paediatric medicines are served up in lurid syrups to make them more palatable to the child, but which have no pharmaceutical value at all. There's often an alternative if you ask.

Commercial BABY FOODS are not made with artificial additives. The one exception is formula milk, which is highly processed in order to change its composition from the cow's milk it is based on which is unsuitable in its natural state. If you want to avoid them in other foods, you'll have to read the labels. And if you want to use colourings in your own food, use vegetable colourings (available from health shops and some supermarkets).

AFTERPAINS

Breastfeeding stimulates the release of the hormone OXYTO-CIN. As well as causing the let-down reflex which makes the breast milk available to the baby, oxytocin helps the uterus to contract, so that it returns to its non-pregnant state. This means that breastfeeding in the early days may be accompanied by contraction-like pains known as afterpains

AIDS

The Aids virus has been found in breast milk, and research so far indicates that at least one baby has contracted the virus through his mother's breast milk. But we really know very little about Aids and its transmission. We don't even know if a baby born with HIV antibodies (because his mother either has Aids, or is already antibody positive and therefore at risk of developing Aids) is better off being breastfed or not. It could well be that breast milk passes on protective qualities that might help the baby fight the disease.

It's a great shame that fear of Aids has caused a few hospitals to close down their milk banks (at least, this has been the official reason given), especially when the Aids virus in breast milk can be totally destroyed with appropriate heat treatment. The majority of milk banks routinely heat-treat donated milk anyway, thus wiping out the risk to any baby receiving the milk.

ALCOHOL

It is the case that alcohol reaches BREAST MILK, although no one has shown that this harms a breastfed baby in any way. Mothers often report that if they have a few glasses of wine at a party, their babies seem to sleep longer! Whether this is actually due to the traces of alcohol in the breast milk is unprovable. But drinking to excess – so that you're actually drunk and incapable – is going to affect your ability to care for the baby, so that's quite obviously not on. A breastfeeding mother who has the occasional drink or two seems at no risk of harming her baby.

ALLERGY

Allergy is an abnormal reaction to any substance – known as an allergen – to which the body has previously been sensitised after first contact. The next time the body meets the allergen, the allergic response is produced, and this can affect just about any part of the body. Typical allergic responses include rashes, watering eyes, diarrhoea, constipation, stomach aches, muscle cramps, lethargy ... Common allergens include foods such as dairy products, wheat, fish, eggs, citrus fruits, house dust, animal fur and soap.

It's now becoming clear that there's a lot more to allergy than was ever dreamed of even 20 years ago. It's known that allergy involves the immune system, and that some conditions are an allergic response rather than an actual disease. This seems particularly so with some cases of ECZEMA and asthma. Some families are more prone to allergy than others because there is a genetic component involved in the development of allergy. If you have a tendency to allergies – not just in terms of food – then it's worth thinking about how you can protect your child against developing allergy herself.

Breastfeeding exclusively for the first six months or so is an important factor – in families with or without allergy. Breast milk doesn't give guaranteed protection against allergy: there's evidence to indicate that susceptible babies can be sensitised to

3

certain things while still in the uterus, and show an allergic response to minute traces of the same substance in their mother's breast milk. However, exclusive breastfeeding definitely helps (that is breastfeeding without top-ups or the odd bottle in the first weeks of life), and so does lengthy breastfeeding (rather than breastfeeding that ends at two or three weeks, or even two or three months). It is believed that breastfeeding allows the body to build up tolerance to foreign substances (ie non-breast milk), working with the body's own immune system in some complex and little-understood way.

A bottle fed baby may be allergic to COW'S MILK – it's known as cow's milk intolerance (see also FOOD INTOLERANCE), and the symptoms seem to be excessive crying, failure to thrive, constant diarrhoea or constipation, rashes and sore bottoms and COLIC. All these symptoms may show up in babies who aren't intolerant, however, which makes the diagnosis a difficult one to reach. If cow's milk intolerance is diagnosed in your baby, you may be prescribed a SOYA MILK formula as a substitute, and this may or may not help. However, it's certainly worth thinking about relactating (starting to breastfeed again) as a means of reducing your baby's symptoms. This can't be done overnight, and it needs motivation and determination, but it can be done (see CHANGING: FROM BOTTLE TO BREAST).

Giving solids early isn't recommended. Four months is early enough for most babies, and if you have allergy in the family, you should put WEANING off for a lot longer – until six months at any rate. Once you give her solids, go slowly on the common allergens (listed above), introduce them in small quantities only and watch for reactions.
See BOOKLIST

ANTIBIOTICS

See MEDICATION AND BREAST MILK

ANTIBODIES

Antibodies are present in the protein immunoglobulin which is carried in the blood. They are essential to the body's immune system – that is, you need them to fight against disease.

Newborn babies are short of antibodies for the first few months, but that doesn't matter if you breastfeed. Breast milk, like blood, has antibodies which are passed on to the baby and used by him to build up his own immunity. GASTROENTERITIS, for example, can be a dangerous disease in a newborn baby, and breast milk gives specific protection against this. Formula milk has none of these anti-infective properties – and therein lies one of its major differences, and disadvantages, compared with breast milk.

APPLE*

An apple is a versatile, enjoyable food that babies can enjoy right from the start of mixed feeding. Choose firm, fresh, unbruised fruit and steer clear of the sharper flavoured varieties at first. Peel, grate and give your baby apple on a spoon, mixed with other foods if you like. Babies older than about six months can have apple as finger food, chopped up into slices or strips. Peel apples until you're sure your baby can cope with them unskinned – probably after a year. Apple makes a quick purée, too (no need to add sugar) and you can vary the texture according to your baby's ability to tolerate lumps.

When? From the first stage of WEANING.

APPLE JUICE

See JUICE

APRICOT*

Apricot can be served as a cooked purée or else well mashed. It also makes good finger food later on. You'll need to peel and stone the apricots you give to your baby, and avoid hard, unripe ones as they can taste sour.

When? From the first stage of WEANING.

AUBERGINE (EGG PLANT)*

The bland flavour of aubergine is especially suitable for babies of all ages. You can cook it by cutting it into slices or chunks, then bring it to the boil and simmer for about ten minutes, or until you can mash it easily. For young babies (up to about seven months) put the mashed-up purée through a sieve, then you'll be able to discard the skin which might be hard to swallow and digest.

When? From the first stage of WEANING.

AVOCADO*

Babies seem to enjoy the smooth taste and texture of avocados. They aren't usually given to babies, mainly, I think, because they still have a faint air of luxury left over from the days when they were an expensive rarity, at least in the UK. These days, however, an avocado may only be a few pennies dearer than an apple. You can mash avocado, uncooked, with a fork, adding enough WATER to make it the consistency you wish. Later, your baby will manage to hold slices and eat it as finger food. It's quite a fatty food, however, so don't introduce it until your baby has become used to a variety of other foods.

When? From the second stage of WEANING.

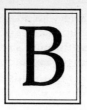

BABY FOODS

I suppose that anything your baby eats or drinks is a 'baby food', but usually the term refers to commercially made formula milk and tins, jars or packets of specially prepared foods designed to be eaten by babies and toddlers, as it does here.

Baby foods are widely available in chemist shops, grocers and supermarkets. There has been something of a tendency to regard them askance over the past few years. I think it's at least partly to do with the suspicion consumers have towards the food industry giants, and the increasing feeling that pre-packaged foods are all 'junk', to be eschewed in favour of fresh foods prepared at home. On the other hand, heavy advertising has also managed to convince some parents that babies *have* to eat baby foods, and that these foods are better than anything that could be made at home – and that's nonsense.

On the whole, though, most parents take a balanced view. I think we're right to be concerned, and critical, about the way commercial interests can affect what we eat or limit the choice of goods available in the shops. However, manufacturers of foods especially made for infants do follow certain production guidelines, which is reassuring. For example, artificial additives and colourings and preservatives are no longer used in these products. It's also true that compared with other pre-packaged foods, baby foods generally have clear information on the outside about the ingredients inside. You can usually tell fairly easily whether sugar is included, or whether the product contains GLUTEN (important for some children with allergies – see ALLERGY). Remember that 'glucose', 'dextrose', 'fructose' and 'sucrose' are all sugars, however.

Baby foods are especially convenient when you're away from home with your child, or when the rest of the family is

7

eating at a different time or having something that isn't very suitable.

There are disadvantages: baby foods are expensive. If a baby is on three commercially packaged meals a day, every day, feeding him will cost several pounds a week. Yet if you feed him on home produced meals only, you hardly notice the blip in your budget, especially if you are already shopping for two adults, or even one. Nutritionally speaking, freshly prepared home cooking, with all the best ingredients, is likely to be better than anything in a tin or packet. However, it is difficult actually to prove that babies on the bought stuff are any less healthy than the others.

Baby foods do tend to be smooth and predictable in their consistency – and even the varieties with lumps in them have a creamy bland texture that just slips down the gullet! Once they're used to this, babies really like it, and become rather stick-in-the-mud about normal foods. In fact, mothers sometimes say their babies get to the stage of being apparently unable to swallow non-smooth food and gag on it, spitting it out rather than chewing and then taking it down. This 'consumer resistance' may also have something to do with the taste of bought baby foods – if you ever sample them yourself, you'll find they just aren't like 'real' food at all, and some toddlers become terribly unadventurous about new tastes and textures. This is never anything more than a temporary problem and eventually a toddler will progress from baby foods, though for some it can take time. It's probably sensible to avoid the situation in the first place by incorporating non-commercial foods in your baby's diet from the start. If you want to avoid commercial baby foods, then it's perfectly possible and healthy to do so. If you prefer to use some, then that's okay, too. And you can mix baby foods with your own – baby rice, for instance, can be used to thicken your own fruit or vegetable purées.

If you do use baby foods when you are first weaning, it makes sense to stick to varieties with only one or two ingredients. That way, if your baby gets a rash, is sick or has any other reaction to his new food you'll have a better chance of pinpointing the offending substance (see also ALLERGY; FOOD INTOLERANCE).

BACON

Very small amounts of bacon used to flavour other foods, such as soup or an omelette, present no problem to a baby eating second stage WEANING foods. Larger quantities are not suitable, however, as bacon is too high in salt for babies and young toddlers.

BANANA*

Weaning can begin with banana, if you like. It's certainly one of the easiest and most nutritious first foods for a baby. It's rich in potassium and vitamins and needs only the minimum preparation. You can make the consistency as smooth or as lumpy as your baby likes by mashing finely or not, and by adding water or milk according to preference. You'll need to boil and cool the water first for a baby under six months, and if you want to use milk to mix, use either expressed breast milk (see EXPRESSING BREAST MILK) or your baby's usual formula milk, made up as you normally would. If your baby has moved onto ordinary full-fat pasteurised milk, this can be used instead. Cut up into slices, bananas make great finger food, too, and older babies can hold a quarter or a half in their hands with enormous enjoyment (and mess, but there we are!). When preparing a banana, cut off as much as you need and then unpeel; the remaining piece will keep for a day or so.

When? From the first stage of WEANING.

BEAN SPROUTS*

Several varieties of pulse or seed can be sprouted to make tiny, crunchy vegetables that can be added as a garnish to other foods or eaten as a side dish. They are an excellent source of protein, vitamins and minerals. You can eat them raw but your baby will find them easier to swallow and digest if they are ground up or cooked first. You can buy sprouts from health and wholefood shops, but they really are easy to grow at home in the kitchen, and you get the benefit of absolute freshness this way.

To grow sprouts, choose from alfalfa, sunflower seeds, soya

9

beans, wheat grains, chickpeas – books on wholefood cookery will give you ideas (untried by me) for other varieties. Wash the pulses well and leave them to soak overnight in a bowl. Drain the next day. Rinse the pulses again and put them at the bottom of a jar (an empty large-size coffee jar is fine), cover the top with a piece of fine cotton cloth, such as muslin, and secure it with string or a rubber band. Keep the jar in a cupboard or a very dark corner for about three days, rinsing and draining the pulses twice each day (three times in hot weather). Don't allow the pulses to sit in the remains of the rinsing water or they will rot so tilt the jar, with the cover on the top, and allow the water to drain out into a bowl. When the sprouts have grown as long as you want them, bring the jar into the light so the leaves can turn green. Rinse them a final time before eating – and eat them within a day.

When? When the second stage of WEANING is well-established.

BEANS & PULSES (dried)*

Butter beans, haricot beans, white beans, kidney beans, lentils, dried peas and split peas are all examples of this category. You normally get the widest variety in wholefood and health stores, but the more popular sorts are available in grocers and super-markets, too.

Babies under six or seven months old *might* find beans and pulses difficult to digest, and even older ones should only have small quantities at a time. Mothers often say beans and pulses give their babies wind pains or make their bowels very active! Your baby may be fine, however, and as always it's best to be guided by him. You need to be especially careful to cook beans and pulses thoroughly. Soak them in cold water for at least six hours or else overnight. Then boil for an hour or an hour and a half until softened (you can use a pressure cooker for this – but remember kidney beans need to be boiled for 20 minutes before being cooked under pressure, this is to neutralise a hard-to-digest acid that is found in them).

All beans and pulses are an excellent source of protein, vitamins and minerals. Once cooked, they can be whizzed up into a paste in a food processor, and served like this or with added water to achieve the consistency you want, or you can

10

sieve or mash them for a less smooth texture. You can also add cooked beans and pulses to soups and stews.

When? From the second stage of WEANING and then in small quantities.

BEEF

See MEAT

BEETROOT

Fresh beetroot can be chopped, puréed or mashed for babies already used to first stage food – it's too fibrous for younger babies even when thoroughly cooked. Cook it in its skin (it needs to simmer in a small amount of water for about an hour) and then peel it before serving. After a meal containing beetroot, you might find your baby's bowel motions take on a red hue, or that bits of beetroot pass straight through undigested. This looks rather startling but it's not significant. Pickled beetroot is not suitable for babies under a year – it's too salty and spicy.

When? From the second stage of WEANING.

BERRIES

Fresh berries – raspberries, strawberries, blackberries, gooseberries and other summer fruits – are easy to prepare and can be used from the second stage of mixed feeding. Berries without tough skins – such as strawberries or blackberries – can be simply washed, hulled and then finely chopped or mashed, or given to a baby as finger food. You can purée or mash the tarter varieties with a naturally sweeter fruit, and fruits like gooseberries with a toughish skin may need to be sieved after cooking, so that you can discard the peel.

When? From the second stage of WEANING.

BIBS

Bibs are essential until your child is well into the toddler stage. If you use terry or muslin nappies, one of these pinned round his neck gives useful protection and enough spare fabric for face and hand wiping as well. Plastic 'pelican' bibs, which catch spills and mess in a turned-up lip, are good and easy to wash up with the rest of the feeding equipment. Many babies dislike the feel of the hard plastic fastening, however, and find these bibs uncomfortable to wear. They prefer the usual towelling or fabric bibs with fabric neck-ties. If you use these, you'll need a clean bib at every mealtime for babies under a year old, so the more you have the better. Bibs with sleeves that are elasticated at the cuff, are good for younger babies who really do get food everywhere, and for babies just learning to feed themselves with a spoon.

BISCUITS*

Of course, biscuits – unless they're free of sugar – can't actually be recommended as a healthy food for babies. They're sweet, they tend to stick to the teeth, and they might fill babies up, to the possible exclusion of other, healthier items. On the other hand, even when trying hard, few parents manage to extend the totally biscuit-free period of a baby's life beyond the first few months of WEANING. Babies enjoy holding them and find them easy to manage; right from the start, they're seen as part of a social occasion when tea, coffee and juice are handed round at toddler groups, mothers' get-togethers and family visits, and let's admit it, a biccie's a quick and convenient baby silencer. But really, if you need to give your baby something, it is far better to offer him a bread stick or a home made rusk.

If you eat a lot of biscuits, do your best to avoid your child doing likewise. However, the occasional biscuit is a harmless treat and feeling guilty about it is pointless. Don't deliberately introduce biscuits to your baby – they're hardly an essential part of a balanced diet, and he's not going to actually want one until he understands that they're nice and that other people like them, and that won't be until about nine months. If you have time, you can make your own biscuits with less sugar than the bought varieties, or even with none.

When? As late as you can get away with!

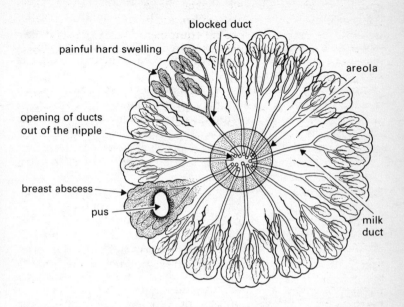

blocked duct

painful hard swelling

areola

opening of ducts
out of the nipple

breast abscess

pus

milk
duct

Diagram of a breast showing the milk ducts leading into the nipple. If a duct becomes blocked a breast abscess may form later.

BLACKBERRIES

See BERRIES

BLENDER/GRINDER

See EQUIPMENT

BLOCKED DUCTS

A blocked duct is a fairly common breastfeeding complication. There are a number of causes, but the effect is basically the same: a small amount of milk gets 'stuck' within one or more milk ducts. Breast milk banks up behind the blockage. The mother can feel a lump in her breast and there seems to be an area of

13

inflammation that shows up as a red patch on the skin, and it's possibly sore. Often, doctors say this is MASTITIS, a breast infection or even a BREAST ABSCESS, and they often advise the mother to stop offering milk from that breast. These diagnoses may be misleading; mastitis means the breast is inflamed and it may not necessarily be infected, and advice to stop feeding is always inappropriate.

Local inflammation does occur round a blocked duct as milk, under pressure, leaks into the bloodstream. The blood recognises the substance as foreign and produces an immune response which results in redness and soreness. The treatment is *not* to stop feeding, this makes the problem worse as it results in further obstructions within the undrained breast, and this can lead to a painful breast abscess.

Instead, massage the affected area as you feed your baby, or as you express. If this is too painful, hot or cold compresses held against the lump will help. The heat improves the circulation of the blood through the breast, and the cold reduces the inflammation – try both and see which works for you. Or else, exercising the arm on the affected side sometimes works, and it's worth changing your feeding position, too. It's also a good idea to check your nipple carefully – sometimes the blockage begins there with what appears to be a fatty plug of milk stopping-up the end of a duct. You might need to squeeze or even pick the 'white spot' out.

If your lump doesn't go in a day or so, after you've tried these measures, then see your doctor. He'll probably prescribe antibiotics which should prevent any true infection from developing (see MEDICATION AND BREAST MILK). You can think about how to prevent the problem happening again by going over what you have, or haven't, been doing. Sometimes a baby may have gone an unusually long time between feeds and this can cause a blockage of undrained milk. Or it may have been a bra that's too tight or ill-fitting, perhaps a 'trap-door' style with a band of elastic round the top of the breast which can put pressure on the ducts. Have you got into the habit of placing your fingers on top of the breast as you feed, perhaps in order to hold your breast away from your baby's nose? (It's better to support your breast from underneath with the flat of your hand if you feel the need to do this). There's speculation that some women may be blessed,

14

or rather plagued, with 'kinked ducts' that are predisposed to blockages or that the whole phenomenon may be linked with allergy, stress or fatigue. A breastfeeding counsellor will be able to discuss other possibilities with you and work out other treatment and means of prevention.
See HELP AND ADVICE

BOTTLE BRUSH

If you're bottle feeding, or if your baby is taking any liquids from a bottle, a special bottle brush helps you clean his bottle efficiently and quickly. It needs STERILISING with other feeding equipment.

BOTTLE FEEDING

Bottle feeding is the process of giving a baby FORMULA MILK in a bottle rather than mother's milk from the breast. On health grounds, bottle feeding is second best to breastfeeding. And there's no point in being equivocal about it – more women would choose to breastfeed and to breastfeed for longer, if they were given fuller information about its benefits and greater help and support when problems arise.

The reasons why most babies in the UK are bottle fed – even if a majority of them begin their lives by being breastfed – are many and I discuss them at various other points in this book. Given that this is the case then it's fortunate that baby formula milks have improved over the last generation or so, and that, in this country, we have the means to feed babies hygienically.

If you decide to bottle feed, don't feel guilty about it. Feeding a baby is a two-way relationship after all, and if *you* feel unhappy about breastfeeding, either from birth, because you haven't found the right help with your feeding problems or because the whole thing has become too much of a struggle, then guilt is inappropriate. Only you know what's right for you and your baby – and you are a unique pair! Most babies thrive satisfactorily on modern formula milk, after all. You may have regrets that breastfeeding didn't work out – but don't feel guilty.

Do choose an appropriate formula for your baby. The days when it was thought that evaporated milk, plus sugar and water,

15

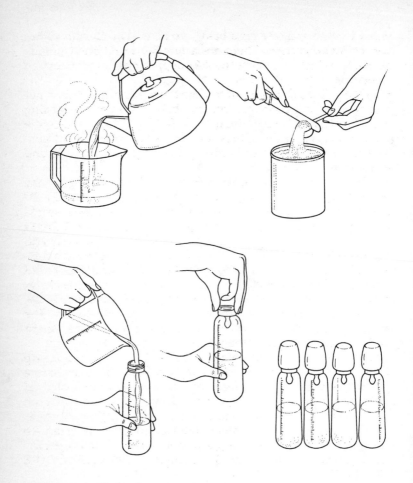

Making up bottle feeds

Make sure that all the equipment is sterilised before you start and wash your hands.

Measure out the water (which should be boiled) straight into the bottle or into a measuring jug, then add the appropriate number of scoops of milk powder (you can level them off with a knife), always reading the instructions carefully. Make sure the powder is fully dissolved.

You can make up single bottles or a full day's feed at one time. This is quite safe as long as you keep it covered in the fridge and don't keep it for more than 24 hours.

16

was adequate and safe for a baby, are gone. Your health visitor will help you choose. There are a number of different brands available which all meet health department guidelines on standards.

STERILISING is important to keep the bottle clean. This is not just because bugs can get into the baby's system via feeding equipment, but also because a bottle fed baby doesn't have the same protection against illness as a breastfed baby and is therefore more susceptible to germs in his bottle, in the teat and elsewhere.

When you're bottle feeding, hold your baby close, and he may need sitting up to be 'winded' every so often (see WIND). Be guided by your health visitor or midwife, and your baby's weight and appetite, as to how much to give him at each feed. Don't force him to finish every last drop every time but tell the health professionals if he always has a poor appetite. Bottle fed babies aren't made to have a rigid routine these days, and they're fed when they seem hungry. In the early days it's very common for this to mean 'little and often', though after the first weeks a bottle fed baby will probably be happy on five or six bottles a day. The amount in those bottles will vary according to the baby's weight and appetite too – you'll soon learn what your baby prefers!

It'll help you to build up a routine in the way you make up feeds. That way, you're less likely to make a mistake. Before giving it to your baby, the feed should be warmed, or cooled, to the right temperature (you test it by shaking a few drops out onto your wrist – it should feel neither warm nor cold). To cool, stand the bottle in a jug of cold water or hold it under a running tap. To warm, stand the bottle in a jug of hot water or use an electric bottle warmer – don't use a microwave (see MICROWAVE COOKING).

Bottle fed babies don't always get the extra comfort from sucking that breastfed babies do; if this makes them fractious, a dummy will help a great deal.

How long should you bottle feed for? Your baby can certainly start using a cup at about five or six months, but there's no reason why you should cut out all his bottles at the same time. In fact, because it takes a while to become proficient with a cup, and most babies will drink smaller amounts from a cup than a bottle anyway, your baby's milk intake may decrease too much if you

17

do this. You can start to reduce his bottles once your baby is taking solids to 'make room' for them (see WEANING). In this society, we tend to disapprove of toddlers running around with bottles, and think they ought to have grown out of the need for them. The way toddlers put their bottles down anywhere and then pick them up again, sometimes much later, probably isn't all that hygienic – another child might take a swig or two, the bottle might fall on the floor and get licked by the cat and so on ... However, many babies enjoy a bottle or two, especially early in the morning and last thing in the evening (to help them get to sleep) at the age of a year and beyond. They do no harm at this age.

Bottles can harm the teeth if your baby is using them for sugary drinks, or even milk, if he goes to sleep with the bottle in his mouth and it remains there. There is also risk of CHOKING. In fact, you shouldn't ever leave a small baby on his own with a bottle propped up on a cushion, as this could cause him to choke, too.

BOTTLES

If you're bottle feeding you'll need at least four feeding bottles; if you're giving only the occasional bottle, one will usually do. Feeding bottles are available in two sizes – designed to hold 100ml or 200ml of fluid (that's about four or eight ounces). They are calibrated so that you can see the amounts marked in five or ten ml sections on the side. The small size is convenient for young babies who don't have large feeds, and for water or juice.

Almost all feeding bottles today are made of a lightweight, clear polycarbonate material, as opposed to glass; they have a wide-neck (unlike older types with a narrow neck). Both these factors make cleaning and STERILISING easier, and the wide neck means milk feeds can be mixed in the bottle.

Some bottles are shaped for supposedly easier gripping, and some have a so called anti-colic design. Some are disposable – you tear off a plastic bottle from a roll, bin-liner fashion, and insert it into a plastic holder. Whatever sort you choose is a matter of personal preference and convenience. I'm totally unconvinced about anti-colic properties, though I suppose they

18

must be worth a try if your bottle fed baby has a problem with COLIC.

Most bottles come complete with a plastic top you screw round the neck which holds the teat and a bottle cover. The cover keeps the bottle clean while it's stored. You can convert some bottles to a feeder cup by substituting the teat for a special, screw-on spouted lid.

BRAS

You don't have to have a special bra while you're breastfeeding, especially if you're naturally small-breasted and don't increase all that much with feeding. If you wear a normal bra, you can slip the cup up or down to allow your baby 'access', but check that the bra doesn't dig into your skin as you feed – it could lead to BLOCKED DUCTS. Many women find their breasts do increase in size during pregnancy and in the first weeks of feeding and then a nursing bra is more comfortable and convenient, even if they go back to an ordinary bra when their breasts 'settle down'.

Nursing bras give good support – important for comfort – and they have some way of opening round the front. The cups may be individually zipped underneath, or they may fasten together with hooks and eyes, a clip or a zip. Alternatively, the bra may have a 'drop cup' which unfastens from the shoulder strap. Bras of this type with an elastic fabric band at the top of the breast aren't recommended, as they can cause blocked ducts as well.

The design of nursing bras has improved in recent years and they are more widely available. The small ads in magazines aimed at young parents and parents-to-be often have information on mail order bras, and the bigger department stores usually have a range in stock. It's a good idea to get measured for a bra, or to send accurate measurements with a mail order. You will normally need two measurements: one taken over the breasts and the other taken under them. Don't buy a nursing bra before you're six or seven months pregnant or you may find you grow out of it! In fact, you're likely to get even larger in the first weeks of feeding, but the adjustable back fastening on most nursing bras can cope with any increase in size.

BREAD*

They call it 'the staff of life', and in our society we certainly eat a lot of it – and a good thing, too. It's a convenient source of carbohydrates, protein and some minerals and vitamins.

Different sorts of bread are becoming more and more widely available, and although generally the bread we buy is made from wheat, bread made from other grains makes a pleasant change for all the family. The best sort of bread to buy is made from the whole of the grain – 'wholemeal', 'wholewheat' or 'wholegrain'. This means that the flour used has undergone less processing, and in particular the outer husk of the grain has been allowed to remain in the milled flour, instead of being discarded. The result is that the bran and valuable B vitamins present in the whole of the grain are all in the bread.

Babies can tolerate small amounts of bread from about six months of age or from the second stage of WEANING.

You can mix small pieces of bread with milk (whatever sort of milk your baby is currently 'on'); use bread or breadcrumbs to thicken soups and purées (pieces of bread whizzed up in the blender or food processor give you the same result); give her 'soldiers' of bread or toast as FINGER FOOD from as early as your baby can manage them. There's no need to cut off crusts unless your baby really can't manage them; many babies like a hardish crust to suck and then chew. Little sandwiches with a light smearing of butter or margarine and made with different fillings are quick and easy, and can even make a balanced meal on their own. Crispbreads are a good alternative, as long as they're not too salty.

Making your own bread isn't difficult, and it's one way of making sure the ingredients are kept simple and wholesome. Shop bread, even the sorts labelled 'free from artificial preservatives', may contain 'extras' to help the bread rise or help the ingredients bind together. It's a lot easier to make your own if you have a freezer, you can make a huge batch of loaves in one or two baking sessions and then store them.

BREAKFAST

Breakfast will be one of your baby's three solid meals a day – when he eventually gets to that stage. You can, to a certain extent, please yourself when you give it to him and if he has a breastfeed, bottle feed or cup of milk first thing in the morning, as many babies do well into toddlerhood, he won't be desperately hungry for an early breakfast. This means that if it suits you to wait until the rest of the household have gone out, you can. On the other hand, you may want to have everybody eating together, and that should be possible too, especially if you give your baby finger food rather than something from a bowl. If you're working, your childminder may be happy to give your baby his breakfast, and that could save valuable time in the morning rush.

Quick and easy breakfasts for under-ones include scrambled or boiled egg (mix with milk to get the right consistency); baby cereal or porridge; other cereals – types which are free of sugar or low in sugar are best and so are the ones you can mash to a pulp with milk as they will be the easiest to manage (like Weetabix or Shreddies); fruit purée. If you have the traditional English fry-up or your partner does, then your baby could have small amounts as long as you have not salted it. Avoid giving him the bacon and sausage, as they are likely to contain too much salt and fat for a baby under a year. Toast is also good at breakfast, either instead of the other suggestions or as well as them. Give it either in small squares or in 'soldier' shapes (ie finger-length oblongs), with a spot of butter or margarine. If you use JAMS AND SPREADS or marmalade those varieties that are free from sugar are best.

BREAST ABSCESS

An abscess is the result of the body's fight against infection. It's a collection of pus – white blood cells that have attempted to engulf the invading infection – that gathers round the affected part. This process can happen within the breast, just as it can happen in a gum, big toe or anywhere in the body. The symptoms are usually as obvious in the breast as elsewhere – redness, swelling, possibly pain. Sometimes pus oozes from the nipple.

A breast abscess is actually fairly rare. Some doctors wrongly call BLOCKED DUCTS or even ENGORGEMENT an abscess, and so you might hear the term more frequently than you should. The abscess always starts with a breast infection – and it rarely develops without obvious symptoms preceding it, as in

21

the case of MASTITIS. The infection can start from a cracked NIPPLE that allows bacteria to get into the breast tissue, or else a germ from the baby's nose. Alternatively, it can begin as a result of an untreated blocked duct, or severe engorgement which leads in its turn to non-infective and then infective mastitis. It's thought that unused milk in the breast creates pressure on the ducts which widen and make it easier for bacteria to enter. If you're told you have a blocked duct or mastitis, it is vital to continue feeding from the affected breast or you will greatly increase your chances of developing an abscess.

Antibiotics are used to treat abscesses, and then surgical drainage if they don't solve the problem quickly enough. You can continue to feed even if you have an abscess, though it may be painful and with a drain in, very difficult (see also MEDICATION AND BREAST MILK).

BREASTFEEDING

Breastfeeding protects your baby against illness, and BREAST-MILK is the most nutritious source of food *and* drink during the first six months of a baby's life; it's convenient, cheap and, for many women and babies, a wonderfully pleasurable experience. So why don't more women in our society choose to breastfeed? And of those that do, why do so many give up after a few days or a few weeks? The health arguments in favour of breastfeeding are very strong and most of us want to do the best we can for our children and worry about whether we're doing the right sorts of things. Surely breastfeeding should be the normal thing to do?

The figures are sobering. In a 1987 survey (see page 232), less than half the women who delivered at a large general hospital in Wales put the baby to the breast *at all*. A London survey published in 1986 (see page 232) reported only 36 per cent of babies still being exclusively breastfed at six weeks. Most people involved in breastfeeding in other parts of the country would say this figure is very high, and that the true national figure is likely to be very much lower. Other western countries – notably Sweden, Denmark, Australia – have far better rates.

I think the reasons for our abysmal breastfeeding situation are complex, but I would identify some of them as follows – not necessarily in order:

• The health benefits of breastfeeding are not stressed by doctors, midwives or health visitors. There's an understandable fear of making non-breastfeeding mothers feel alienated or guilty, but as a result you could be forgiven for not thinking that it mattered all that much.

• Until now, there's never been a government-sponsored campaign to encourage breastfeeding and underline its advantages.

• Health professionals are not adequately trained in helping mothers overcome even the most basic breastfeeding problems (many women stop breastfeeding because they have real physical problems with it). Problems which are initially slight are allowed to get worse and worse, until even highly-motivated women give up in despair.

• Women themselves are not very well-informed about breastfeeding, and don't know where to go for the right sort of help if they have questions or problems.

• Our society is hung-up about breasts and sexuality. Women (and not only younger women, although they are especially unlikely to breastfeed and likely to be less than entirely at home with their own bodies), are sometimes reluctant, even embarrassed to breastfeed at all, and those feelings are intensified if they have to do it in front of other people. You can't shut yourself away if you're breastfeeding – and why should you?

• Men (partners and dads) may find it difficult to 'share' a woman's breasts with a baby and may undermine the notion of breastfeeding as a result. If you're breastfeeding six, seven or eight (or more) times a day, you are going to encounter adverse comments and hostility is going to be a frequent problem.

• The promotion of bottled formula milk has been allowed to go on far too much in this country. The Food Manufacturers Federation has been allowed to adopt a different code of practice from the World Health Organisation's code on breast milk substitutes. The WHO CODE outlawed many of the commercial practices that had been shown to promote bottle feeding at the expense of breastfeeding. Among the clauses which are missing, or have been considerably altered, in the FMF code are the ones that ban the advertising of formula milk and all its attendant paraphernalia. Those which deal with free product samples for new mothers, and the ones which refer to the way breast milk substitutes are packaged have now been acknowledged.

23

There are other reasons, and each woman is likely to have her own special set of circumstances and feelings which she takes into account when she decides how she is going to feed her baby. I don't think the fact that more women may go out to work part-time or full-time when their babies are still small has very much to do with the situation, except occasionally. Few women return in the first four months, and those that do tend to be in skilled or professional jobs and they are more likely to breastfeed anyway. The women I meet in this situation often continue to breastfeed, or breast and bottle feed, with great success.

The question of class is fascinating. Why are middle class women more likely to breastfeed? Also the further north you travel through England and Scotland, breastfeeding rates can be seen to decline. Is this tied up with class as well? And exactly how important are hospital practices in establishing breastfeeding? What about the antenatal period – could more information be given?

You'll have guessed from this that I'm in favour of more women breastfeeding! But I don't think anyone should be forced into it, or persuaded against their will. I do think that given the right atmosphere in society, the correct information, the right support and, most important of all, effective help with problems, most women would choose to breastfeed. It's estimated that 95 per cent of women are physically capable of breastfeeding. In practice, too many of us are sold short by our anti-breastfeeding culture. The irony is that some women who do switch from the breast to the bottle report that their babies are happier and 'more settled'. This is often the case where a women has had a problem with her MILK SUPPLY and hasn't been able to increase it, usually because of poor advice and lack of encouragement.

Babies whose mothers have decided they really don't want to breastfeed for whatever reason, are probably better off on the bottle. Why spoil your relationship because of resentment about your feeding method? If you're taking medication for some chronic condition, such as epilepsy or asthma, then check with your doctor that it's okay to breastfeed. Don't take 'no' for an answer – there may be alternative drugs available, or there may even be ways of fitting in feeds round your doses and working out when trace amounts are likely to have disappeared from the milk (see also MEDICATION AND BREAST MILK). If breastfeeding has become a struggle because of the way your life has changed, or because of problems that you can't resolve and there's no chink of light at the end of the tunnel, then only you can decide the moment to call it a day, and really start to enjoy being a mum.

Sometimes, full breastfeeding isn't possible because of illness – mother's or baby's – which means mother and baby are separated. However, EXPRESSING BREAST MILK may cope with this. Defects in the baby's mouth, such as a CLEFT LIP AND/OR PALATE, may make breast feeding very difficult, and sometimes impossible. HANDICAPPED BABIES or babies with congenital disabilities, such as a heart defect, are hard to breastfeed. A PRE-TERM BABY may need to be fed by a nasogastric tube which takes food through the nose to the stomach. It is always more difficult to breastfeed in these circumstances, but with support and patience it can be done. Finally, it does seem that a very few women, for reasons we don't yet understand, do find it impossible to build up enough milk to feed their babies exclusively on breast milk – no matter what they do.

There are then, and there always will be, physical and social factors to prevent every mother feeding her baby on her breast milk alone for the first six months. In any case, it would be wrong to make anyone feel bad about their method of feeding. Mothers need more ego-boosting, not less! So don't let anyone or anything, least of all this book, make you feel guilty if you bottle feed. You may have regrets – we all do about something we've done when our children were small – and you may feel angry that the right sort of help isn't or wasn't available to you, but bottle feeding doesn't mean you're any worse or better a mother than anyone else.

It's only fair to state the positive feelings about breastfeeding and to acknowledge the 'nice bits' about it, over and above the health benefits. When breastfeeding goes well, it can be very fulfilling, calming and relaxing; the knowledge that you and your body are responsible for the growth and health of your baby is both awe-inspiring and gratifying. If you're in two minds about whether to have a try, then at least give it a go. It's always easier to make the switch to the bottle if you decide it's not for you, than the other way round.

See USEFUL ADDRESSES.

How it works Your breasts prepare for breastfeeding just as soon as you're pregnant, in fact, many women notice a tingling sensation or extra sensitivity in their breasts before they miss their first period. Already, the breasts are forming the tissue they will need to make and store milk for the baby. At some time in the first two months of pregnancy you'll notice MONT-GOMERY'S TUBERCLES on the nipple. They are not so obvious if you've been pregnant before as once formed they never entirely go away. These are the tiny exit points belonging to the sebaceous glands that keep the nipple soft and supple. Throughout pregnancy, your breasts will feel and look larger than usual, and you might find it more comfortable to wear a bra. You produce COLOSTRUM in pregnancy – a creamy yellow fluid that precedes the production of breast milk – and you may find that it leaks out. But, once your baby's born, the hormone PROLACTIN starts to circulate in your bloodstream, and it's this that stimulates the production of milk. Breast milk is made from nutrients in the blood, and it's interesting to note that this means you have a very similar nutritional relationship with your baby when you're breastfeeding to the one you had when you were pregnant; throughout that time, nutrients from your blood were synthesised by the placenta, and then transferred to the baby via the blood stream in the umbilical cord.

Milk is made and stored in the breasts, in 20 or so lobes, and milk ducts lead from the lobes to the nipple. Just behind the nipple are tiny reservoirs where a small amount of milk can be stored, but the bulk of the milk is further away, inside the breast. At some time between the second and fifth day after delivery, your milk 'comes in' – that means the breasts now produce milk instead of colostrum. You may notice your breasts feel and look full, not just as a result of more milk, but also because the breasts have a greatly increased blood supply at this time and tissue fluids increase in volume as well. However, this isn't always very noticeable, especially if your baby is already sucking frequently as this seems to facilitate the transition. If you don't put your baby to the breast, this milk will dwindle away, although it might be uncomfortable for a day or so. It's only by feeding your baby that you'll maintain your MILK SUPPLY, as it's the feeding that causes the production to be stimulated. Feeding your baby causes two hormonal responses – prolactin, which 'tells' the body to make more milk, and OXYTOCIN, which causes tiny muscles in the milk-storing lobes to release the milk. This is the LET-DOWN REFLEX and it allows the milk to go down the milk ducts towards the nipple . . . and from there into your baby.

One basic fact about breastfeeding that's important to remember is that the more you feed, the more milk you'll produce. This is why it's possible for mothers to feed TWINS and even triplets, because twice or three times the stimulation means twice or three times the milk (that's not to minimise the organisational and physical problems sometimes involved in feeding more than one baby. It is also more difficult for women to build up such an abundant supply). So establishing and maintaining a good milk supply usually means frequent feeding at first – feeding as and when your baby needs it (he'll tell you by waking and crying). This is known as 'DEMAND FEEDING' or 'feeding on demand'. I don't like either of these expressions as both of them conjure up the image of a tiny demon imperiously ordering you to feed him! The alternative expression, 'ask feeding' is also unconvincing. Instead, I prefer 'unrestricted feeding', the phrase used by Doctors Andrew and Penny Stanway in *Breast is Best* (see BOOKLIST). If you have a SLEEPY BABY who doesn't 'demand' to be fed by being restless and/or crying, and seems to prefer to sleep instead of waking for feeds, then wake him and feed him anyway – don't let him go more than three hours between feeds. Feed him whenever you want to or whenever he appears wakeful, even if he isn't actually crying. We can sometimes be reluctant to feed a baby when he wants to be fed. People might tell you that you're spoiling your baby, or that he'll never get into a routine. It's essential to remember that a tiny baby's wants are the same as his needs. Feeding him won't spoil him although, yes, he enjoys feeding and may enjoy the experience of sucking just as much as he enjoys the feeling of a full tummy. He may be hungry sooner and more irregularly than a bottle fed baby, but that's because breast milk may be digested more quickly than formula milk *and* because he may take varying amounts of milk at each feed, in tune with his appetite. Some experts think that this natural appetite control, learnt at the breast rather than the experience of being encouraged to finish a bottle, may help with weight control later in life.

For the first couple of days after birth, many babies are sleepy, and just not apparently hungry. They only start to need frequent feeds when the milk comes in. A baby of two to three weeks is likely to feed several times a day and night. It is misleading to put a number on it as some of the 'feeds' may be very short or the end of one feed may merge with the beginning of another, especially in the evenings. However, it's unlikely to be less than eight times, and may be more. As your baby gets older he'll be able to space his feeds out as he becomes able to hold more milk in his tummy; he can suck more efficiently and you produce more milk each time. It is possible to work towards ROUTINES if that suits you best, and once the milk supply is established, it needs less frequent stimulation. But in the early weeks, take a cue from your baby as to the best way to get LACTATION underway.

Bottles of formula milk confuse the milk supply. Your body doesn't get the message to produce more milk, and produces less. In addition to that, the baby may stay asleep – and therefore not feeding – for longer because of the length of time needed to digest some formulas. So, COMPLEMENTARY AND SUP-PLEMENTARY BOTTLES (or 'comps' or 'top-ups') are bad news for breastfeeding, especially in those vulnerable early weeks. They make a problem with milk supply worse, not better. If you're keen to breastfeed you'll avoid them.

The emotional responses of breastfeeding   Of course, feeding your baby isn't just a way of filling her up to keep her healthy and make her grow. It's a special way of demonstrating your care, and of showing you love her. This is true whether or not you choose to breastfeed. Babies, on the whole, enjoy feeding, and it's rewarding for you, too, to watch their pleasure and content-ment. Many women positively enjoy breastfeeding. It's such a pleasurable thing to do when it's going well, indeed, one of the hormonal effects of breastfeeding is to relax you. For some, these feelings may occasionally be sexually arousing, though far more often, they simply allow you to feel soothed and calmed. It's also enormously satisfying to see your baby growing each week, and to watch her development, knowing it's 'all my own work'. Breastfeeding is a very loving, very 'womanly' thing to do, and something you'll look back on with fondness years after you have weaned.

Feelings of rejection are sometimes experienced by women

who find their babies are 'difficult' feeders and perhaps experience BREAST REFUSAL. This is understandable – there you are, possibly feeling emotionally raw after childbirth, ready and willing to give him what you know is best, and he seems either indifferent or hostile to the idea. Please don't feel rejected by your baby. Bear in mind that he doesn't come into the world knowing that babies ought to love their mothers. He enjoys the feelings of security and comfort you give him, but as for actually loving you – well, that comes later. All he needs is skilled help in getting at the milk in your breasts. He's not rejecting you; he's just expressing annoyance at the fact that his tummy isn't being filled, and frustrated at not being able to fill it.

Later on, women whose babies go through the process of WEANING themselves by suddenly rejecting the breast – and continuing to reject it – may feel hurt. Or, weaning may take place gradually and untraumatically, but you may still feel regret at the way that chapter of your life has closed. All these experiences are growing and learning ones. It's natural to feel sadness that a relationship you have enjoyed is going to be expressed in ways other than feeding – but you will get over this. Some of the sadness may even be connected to the physical effect of hormones in retreat as breastfeeding comes to an end. When your body stops producing milk, your feelings may be easier to cope with.

BREASTFEEDING COUNSELLOR

See HELP AND ADVICE

BREAST MILK

Breast milk is the perfect food and drink for baby humans, for at least the first four to six months of life. We now know that it has yet to be fully analysed, as the boffins keep discovering previously unrecognised components.

We've known for a while that breast milk contains ANTIBODIES which protect the baby from many illnesses. And we're just beginning to appreciate how well breast milk adapts to the changing needs of the baby as it grows. For example, the milk a baby takes in his first weeks is more concentrated in calories than the milk he'll take at, say, four months. The mother of a PRE-TERM BABY produces a different kind of milk, particularly suited in mineral and vitamin content to her baby at this time.

It's also been shown that the composition of breast milk may change from feed to feed, and it seems quite clear that it is meant to be adaptable. The FORE MILK – the milk the baby receives at the start of the feed – is more watery than the fattier HIND MILK which he receives later on. In all these respects, breast milk differs from formula milk, which is the same at every feed, and throughout every feed, for every baby.

Can breast milk vary in quality? Generally speaking, the evidence is that mothers have to be severely malnourished and living under virtually famine conditions before the quality of their milk is affected, although there hasn't been a great deal of reliable research on western women. Quantity is more likely to suffer. However, the baby may be sensitive to the traces of his mother's diet which may be found in breast milk. So if your baby seems unhappy or is prone to COLIC it may well be worth thinking about what you eat, while making sure you don't go short of nutrients yourself. If you need medication, tell your doctor you are breastfeeding and he'll make sure anything you take is considered safe. Some drugs, such as those taken for asthma or epilepsy, may be harmful to the baby as they are secreted into breast milk. You need to get up-to-date and accurate information from your doctor about the advisability of breastfeeding while taking them (see also MEDICATION AND BREAST MILK).

BREAST PADS

See LEAKING FROM BREASTS

BREAST PUMPS

If you are EXPRESSING BREAST MILK for any reason, you can either do it by hand or with a pump. These can be either electrically operated (battery or mains) or else operated manually. Different women prefer different pumps and it's hard to predict exactly which sort will suit you.

Electrical pumps that work from the mains are very bulky, and

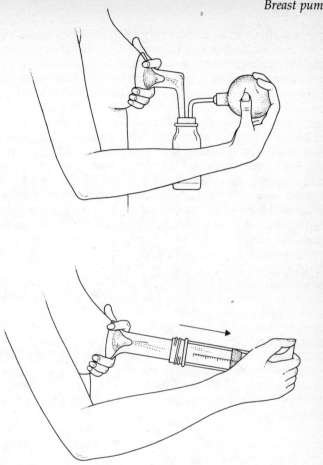

Two examples of hand pumps.

far too expensive for most mothers to contemplate actually buying (something like £500). However, you can hire one from local branches of the National Childbirth Trust, who have agents in many areas (see USEFUL ADDRESSES). In some places, pumps may be available on free loan for mothers who cannot afford the hire charges. Battery operated pumps are a lot cheaper (about £40), far smaller and more convenient. It's probably only worthwhile going to the expense of hiring or buying an electric pump if you intend to use it frequently, perhaps because your baby cannot feed from the breast (because he's too ill, or because you're separated from him for some reason). Hand pumps are cheap (about £8) and they are light and easy to carry about. The most popular types work on a reverse bicycle pump principle, and they convert to a feeding bottle. This sounds a boon, but it may not be of any use to you as you may want to actually store the milk instead of using it straight away. If you store it in the bottle/pump you won't be able to use it to express in the meantime. One other sort of pump is known as a breast reliever, and costs about £4. This is fine for relieving the pressure of ENGORGEMENT, but it can't be recommended for collecting breast milk to use, as sterilising the pump cannot be adequately ensured.

BREAST REFUSAL

When a baby seems to resist the breast it is known as breast refusal. The baby may refuse to open his mouth to grasp the nipple, he may cry and turn his face away, he may actually push the breast away with his hands, he may start to feed and then come off, crying, after only a short time ... it only needs to happen a few times, and both mother and baby can be greatly upset. Breast refusal is by no means a permanent refusal in every case, and if you're keen to carry on breastfeeding don't feel your baby's rejected the whole thing.

In a new baby, breast refusal may simply be caused by sleepiness and exhaustion – maybe after a long and tiring labour, perhaps as a result of drugs the mother was given, perhaps because of neonatal JAUNDICE or because the baby is premature, or 'light-for-dates' (underweight for his age). In many cases, there seems to be no obvious reason why the baby seems less than enthusiastic about getting started with breastfeeding. You just need patience, understanding from those around you and some help in making sure that your baby is LATCHING ON properly. It *can* take a little while for breastfeeding – a learning process – to become easy for the two of you. Later on, breast refusal can be caused by the simple fact that the baby isn't hungry. Not all babies like to suck for the sake of it; some just want to sleep, sit up and look around, or lie in your arms without feeding. If he doesn't seem to be interested in the second breast, just feed from the 'unused' side first next time. (One-sided feeding is something most babies do from time-to-time; a few seem to only need one side at almost every feed. It doesn't matter as long as your baby is thriving and happy.)

Breast refusal can happen as a result of the baby being given COMPLEMENTARY AND SUPPLEMENTARY BOTTLES, and so the baby protests at the breast and only settles down to feed once a bottle is given. The reasons for this may be complex: the baby gets used to having his milk lying on his back, and resents the way he can't look around when on the breast; he starts to dislike the waiting time between sucking and getting the full flow of breast milk, and this waiting time may have increased because the mother's LET-DOWN REFLEX isn't working very well; or the MILK SUPPLY has decreased with the use of bottles, and the baby protests at the slow flow. Interestingly, babies who are bottle fed while their mothers are at work, and who are breastfed when their mothers return, don't seem to refuse the breast. Why is this? Because the bottles are given quite separately from the breastfeeds, and moreover, they aren't given by the mother – so the baby knows there's no bottle to come after the breast? Nobody really knows.

I have known babies to start refusing the breast when MEN-STRUATION restarts. Or the mother has had an excess of some unusual food although how the baby recognises and responds to this we don't know. It may be that taste plays a part in breast-feeding, and menstruation and unusual foods actually make the milk taste different. Medication, going on the Pill, the use of perfume or sprays near the nipple – all these can cause breast refusal (see also CONTRACEPTION; MEDICATION AND BREASTFEEDING). Babies who have colds or blocked noses find it hard to suck as it's difficult to breathe while feeding, so they may also fight at the breast. Try a baby's menthol rub (from the chemist) to help with this. Sick babies sometimes feed poorly and so a medical check is needed. TEETHING babies may not want to suck because perhaps it's painful on their gums, who knows? But a bit of teething gel applied just before the feed can often have a dramatic effect, so it's worth a try, even if you can't see any signs of teeth coming through. Some babies just give up the breast at five, six or seven months for no apparent reason, but if this happens to you, it is best to think about whether any of the above factors could be contributing.

If you can identify a reason for breast refusal, then this will help you solve the problem. If bottles are contributing to it, then try to phase them out (with a breastfeeding counsellor's or health visitor's support). Give fewer solids if your baby's on mixed feeding. If you can't identify a reason, and even if you can, be patient; continue to offer your baby the breast at your usual times; in addition, pick moments when he's sleepy and less likely to resist the lure of a gentle, calming suck! You may need to find a quiet space, away from distractions. If you start suffering from ENGORGEMENT with the sudden lessening of demand on your milk supply, then try EXPRESSING BREAST MILK to keep comfortable. Don't worry about your milk dwindling through lack of stimulation – if this does happen it will return when your baby gets back onto the breast.

BREAST SHELLS/SHIELDS

Breast shells or shields are plastic cones worn over the nipple, and their most important function is to draw out flat or inverted nipples in preparation for feeding. It's true that babies may have problems LATCHING ON to flat or inverted nipples, and shells may improve the shape. But I have seen no study that indicates that women who wear shells during their pregnancy do any better at feeding than women who don't, however. Nipples improve in shape during pregnancy and the early weeks of feeding anyway. It might be worth trying the shells, nevertheless. Don't wear them for long – you can get sweaty and soggy inside and the nipples can actually become sore and crack. There's no absolute time limit, but two hours at a time in pregnancy, or, after your baby's born, half an hour before you expect to feed, seem sensible guidelines. Some women who 'leak' breast milk use the shells to collect the drops between feeds, but the shells can actually encourage leaking in themselves.

See LEAKING FROM BREASTS

BREASTS – SIZE OF

Large breasts, small breasts, medium breasts – we're all different, and the size of your breasts won't affect breastfeeding in the slightest. Most women find their breasts get larger during pregnancy, and for the first six weeks or so of breastfeeding. They then seem to settle down a little, and you don't get the enlargening and softening before and after a feed you may have observed before. It can take several months, even as long as two years, after breastfeeding has stopped for the glandular tissue of the lactating breast to be replaced by fat, and it's fat that gives the breast its shape. You may feel a bit 'floppy' in the meantime.

BROCCOLI*

Rich in iron and vitamins, broccoli is becoming more widely available and as it's quick to cook and easy to mash, so it's a useful vegetable for a baby. Don't use too much water when you cook it or it will end up looking sloppy and dispirited! Broccoli can steam in a small amount of liquid on a low heat – it takes about ten minutes, depending on how finely chopped it is and how much you have.

When? From the second stage of WEANING.

BUTTER

Because of the bad press dairy products and foods high in fat have received recently, you could be forgiven for assuming your baby ought to totally avoid butter. However, butter is a useful source of fat and vitamins and as long as it's spread in small quantities it's not harmful. Margarines which are high in polyunsaturates are a better alternative to butter, however, as a general rule.

When? From the second stage of WEANING.

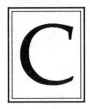

CABBAGE*

There's a good variety of cabbage available these days, all suitable for a baby as long as the texture's right for his age. It's a good source of iron, calcium and vitamins. Chop and cook in the usual way, using as little water as possible. Your baby can have raw white (Dutch) cabbage, or red cabbage, in a salad, as long as the pieces are chopped up or grated very finely although avoid this with young babies as they might find it hard work to digest. Try mixing cooked or raw cabbage with other simply prepared foods, such as apple, or small slivers of cooked or blanched onion (for babies over nine months).

When? Cooked, from the second stage of WEANING. Raw, finely chopped, from nine months.

CAFFEINE

If you're breastfeeding, and you drink more than half-a-dozen drinks of tea, coffee or cola a day – all of which contain caffeine – then your baby may show the effects of this by being restless and difficult to settle. Caffeine gets through to the breast milk, and seems to 'wind the baby up' in this way. You'll need to cut out caffeine completely for a few days to make a difference, and to work out whether your baby is being affected. Drink decaffeinated coffee instead, or herbal teas and fruit juices.

CAKE*

Cake is hardly an essential item of anyone's diet, and if you're keen to avoid sugar, you can certainly keep it out of your child's diet for quite some time before he knows what he's missing.

Compromises could include making cakes low in sugar, or sugar-free. Babies can cope with most sorts of cake from about six months, though you shouldn't give a baby cake with large pieces of nut or whole nuts, because of the risk of CHOKING.

CALCIUM

Calcium is one of the essential minerals needed in every human being's diet. Its functions include the development of bones and teeth, and to keep them healthy. It's present in dairy products, eggs, some green vegetables and some fish. It's also in breast milk and formula milk, though the levels in formula milk have had to be artificially lowered from the high levels present in unmodified cow's milk.

CALORIES

It's more correct to refer to kilocalories or K-calories – though it's acceptable to use the term Calories, with a capital 'C'. In dietary terms, a Calorie measures a unit of energy. The body needs to metabolise a food to function normally. Food is described as 'containing' Calories, and people are described as 'needing' a certain amount of Calories in order to function normally, and, in the case of babies and children, in order to grow.

A baby under about six months needs approximately 500 to 700 Calories a day. From six months to a year, his needs increase to about 950 Calories a day. You don't ever need to actually count your baby's Calories, however. Your breast milk (or formula, if you're bottle feeding) will supply all the Calories your baby needs for at least the first four to six months, and when you begin WEANING, it's fine to go gradually and allow your common sense and your baby's appetite to help you judge the amounts he should have.

When you're breastfeeding, *you* need extra Calories in order to make the milk. If the total number of Calories in the milk that you give to your baby equals 500 to 700 a day, you'd think that was the amount you yourself need to take in, but, in fact, research indicates that you only actually need about half of this because the body uses energy so much more efficiently at this time. However, many women do find that they are hungrier when they're breastfeeding, especially at first, and this could be the body's way of letting you know when extra food is needed. Eat according to your appetite when you're breastfeeding – but eat sensibly (see also DIET AND BREASTFEEDING).

CARBOHYDRATE

A carbohydrate is a combination of carbon, hydrogen and oxygen, to speak scientifically, and carbohydrates are most easily recognised in sugars and starches. They're the main source of energy for the body. Unrefined carbohydrates have their full amount of vitamins, minerals and dietary fibre, and they're therefore more nutritious than refined carbohydrates. Good examples include brown or wholegrain flour (a starch) and products made from it.

CAROB POWDER*

Carob powder is a powder extracted from the carob bean. It has a pleasant, chocolate-like flavour, and it's often used as an alternative to CHOCOLATE in wholefood cooking. It's a source of iron, and is useful for people who are sensitive to chocolate.

CARROTS*

Carrots are a great favourite with many babies, probably because the taste is naturally sweet, without being strong in flavour, and I expect they like the colour, too! Cook them like other vegetables – scraping, chopping and then boiling in a minimal amount of water – and then cut up, mash or purée. If you're using old carrots, you should peel them finely first. Cook sticks of carrot, and your baby can hold them as 'finger food' from the age of about six or seven months. Raw carrot, grated finely and then chopped, can be managed by older babies in small quantities. Some babies like carrot juice, though you need to dilute it well if you're making your own or it will be too strong.

When? From the first stage of WEANING. Raw carrot: small, finely grated pieces from about nine months.

38

CASSEROLES*

A casserole is normally a one-pot dish of vegetables and meat, cooked in an oven. It's probably rather a waste of time and effort to make a casserole especially for a baby – the quantity for one meal is rather small. However, a casserole made for him at the same time as you make one for the rest of the family is a practical alternative. You can put salt and seasoning in the larger one as well as those ingredients you don't want to give your baby, and put the junior version in a separate vessel, cooking it at the same time. Or, if you're happy with the contents, leave the whole casserole unseasoned until you actually serve it. Just extract your baby's portion and serve it to him without seasoning, chopping it so it's a suitable texture. In this way, if you eat a lot of casseroles (and they're certainly good value and practical) your baby can join in your meals well before the end of his first year. Remember that the fact that you'll tend to offer several foods in one go when you give your baby a casserole means that it's best to wait until she is already used to a variety of different foods.

When? From about six to eight months, depending on how quickly you take the pace of mixed feeding and depending on the ingredients of the dish (see also WEANING).

CAULIFLOWER*

Cauliflower is a vegetable that babies enjoy on the whole. You can serve the cooked leaves and stem as well as the creamy-coloured flowers, but first discard any discoloured or damaged leaves, and make sure you wash it well after chopping it up. Purée, chop or mash after cooking, and later small cooked pieces make excellent finger food. You can serve tiny pieces raw to an older baby.

When? From the first stage of WEANING. Raw (in very small pieces) from about nine months.

CELERY*

Prepare celery like other vegetables. You can serve the leaves as well as the stalk. Babies can't cope with raw celery, and won't until they have enough teeth to chew through it, before then they might break off a piece and then there's a danger of CHOKING.

When? From the second stage of WEANING.

CEREALS*

Cereals are a source of carbohydrate, fibre, protein, minerals and vitamins, as well as being low in fat, and in most parts of the world cereal or cereals, of some sort, are an important part of the daily diet. In this country we eat a lot of wheat in different forms but there's a good variety of other cereals available these days, so you don't have to stick to the same sorts – or reserve it for breakfast, only, either.

Young babies, under six months, should have refined cereals at first. Whole grains, although they are more complete nutritionally, are more fibrous and more difficult to digest. If you do use unrefined cereals make sure that they're well cooked. As your baby gets older, he'll be able to cope with unrefined cereals, though it's still best to go gradually with them, and watch for your baby's reaction, if any. A further reason for going slowly with whole grains is that a baby whose diet is still based almost entirely on milk, and this should apply to the majority of babies under six months, is likely to 'fill up' very quickly, leaving less room in his tummy for what is still the ideal food at his age: breast milk (or formula milk). In fact, this tummy-filling quality of cereal, whether it is refined or unrefined, is a point to watch; it's actually quite easy to give too much too early. Giving cereal in a bottle used to be common but we know now that this is inadvisable. It's overloading a baby as he may glug the whole lot down because it's an easy way to eat, and you're even running the risk of DEHYDRATION because he won't get enough fluid this way. Don't give GLUTEN to a young baby (under six months). Gluten is a protein found in certain cereals – including wheat, rye, barley and oats – and ALLERGY or signs of FOOD INTOLERANCE as a result of it, are symptoms of COELIAC DISEASE. If you have allergy in the family, then stick to gluten-free cereals until your baby is at least eight or nine months old, and therefore better able to tolerate the protein. Wheat itself is also frequently implicated in cases of food allergy, without the sensitivity being related to the gluten in it, so if you're worried about allergy that's another reason for delaying the introduction of wheat – in whatever form.

So, what is a good age to think about cereals, and what sort should your baby have at what age? If your baby's starting on mixed feeding, then cereal is one sort of food you can start off with. Stick to a gluten-free, refined cereal like short-grain white RICE or white rice flakes. Alternatively, you can buy one of the branded baby cereals which are normally rice-based (check the ingredients on the packet). These are usually fortified with vitamins and minerals – you don't need the sort fortified with sugar in any form. A baby still mostly on breast milk or formula milk doesn't really need the vitamins and minerals added to the baby rice either, but the advantage of the packets is that they're convenient; you can mix them quickly, and it's not fiddly or time-consuming to make up tiny quantities. You don't have to mix the baby rice with formula or breast milk. You can use water (previously boiled and cooled for a young baby) or the juice from cooking vegetables or fruit. Other gluten-free cereals include millet and maize, which are not so easy to find as rice, though health food shops will stock some of them, at least. Once your baby's used to this sort of cereal, he can progress to others, and to foods with different cereals in them (providing he's at least six months, and older if you have allergy in the family). Don't stick to the obvious: you can make porridge with millet instead, for instance. And cereals can be very useful as a basis for other foods – the bland taste of rice, for instance, mixes well with fruit and vegetables. You can thicken soups and sauces with cereal until they are the right texture for your baby, or add them to casseroles and stews.

See WEANING

CHANGING

From bottle to breast Changing from bottle to breast can be done, and it's known as relactation. You do need to be highly motivated and to have a lot of patience because it's rarely very easy or quick to do. You may decide you want to breastfeed your child because you regret that you started bottle feeding – maybe you never actually got started with breastfeeding, or perhaps you started and then switched to the bottle because of difficulties. Once a woman has had a baby, she produces breast milk, but the production line shuts down if there are no demands made upon it. However, it can be started up again with sufficient stimulation – and this is why you hear tales of grandmothers in the Third World breastfeeding their daughter's babies, years after their last child was born. For us, in this society, the experience of relactation will be mainly confined to babies who have got used to the bottle – and that adds a difficulty to the whole process. It's true that the sooner you decide to relactate, the easier it seems to be. If it's just a matter of days after switching, your breasts will need less stimulation before responding, and your baby has had correspondingly less time to become 'stuck' on the bottle. Leave it a month or two and your body needs more stimulation to get things going, but your baby is even less inclined to change; he may have forgotten how to suck on the nipple and may get very impatient and distressed when his food doesn't come. Those are the physical facts about relactating, but there are other facts about the benefits of breast milk which you may feel are persuasive enough to motivate you to try overcoming any difficulties. If you feel upset and guilty about giving up breastfeeding, then successful relactation may help you, too. On the other hand, you have to think about what you'd feel if you *don't* manage it, or if the whole thing develops into a stressful, anxious challenge ... A breastfeeding counsellor, or a sympathetic and informative health visitor or midwife, will help you make up your mind – and will give you encouragement and support whatever you decide (see HELP AND ADVICE).

Start by putting your baby to your breast as often as you can – or as often as he'll accept it. He may go to the breast happily, but make a dreadful fuss if he finds there's nothing there. In this situation, you might be best giving him his bottle first, and then allowing him to suck when he's partially or fully satisfied. Some mothers have found their babies respond best to the breast when they're already a little sleepy, and they can enjoy a 'comfort suck'. This encourages the baby to take pleasure in returning to the breast, and it stimulates the supply as well. Try EXPRESSING BREAST MILK either by hand or with a BREAST PUMP, as this will stimulate your supply as well. You may need to cut down on your baby's bottles very gradually. Be guided by his appetite. However, once you feel you have milk in your breasts again, you'll have the confidence *not* to satisfy your baby's hunger with formula milk at every feed. You may be able to give an ounce or two less at some feeds, and work up to missing out the occasional bottle and giving 'breast only'. Ask your breastfeeding counsellor about a feeding device, sometimes known as a Lact-Aid, Supply-Line or a nursing supplementer. This has a tube attached to a bag, which you fill with formula milk. The end of the tube is placed near the nipple, with the rest of the tube going round your neck and the bag resting on your chest. The idea is that the baby takes both tube and nipple into his mouth, and sucks on both. He gets rewarded with food for his sucking as the formula milk is drawn up through the tube and this satisfies his hunger. At the same time, the nipple is receiving direct stimulation. The process is designed to lead to the breast gradually taking over, or at least permanently supplementing the formula feeding. There are some encouraging reports of successful relactation with a supplementer, but it *is* fiddly to use and STERILISATION is difficult. You need a lot of determination to persevere with it. Some babies don't get the hang of fixing on to the tube and nipple, and become exhausted and cross when the mum tries to insist.

Mothers who have relactated successfully are always convinced it was worth it. Some are suprised that although they were prepared for problems, they managed it in such a short time after all. So if you have the time and the motivation, and the emotional support from those around you, relactating could well be a serious option.

From breast to bottle   There are situations when this is the right thing to do. It's much better if *you* decide it's right for you – being pressurised into a decision to switch can lead to anger and unhappiness. It is so easy to change from breastfeeding to BOTTLEFEEDING yet it's a big step to take, because it's not so easy to change back (as we've seen, above). Remember that if you don't *want* to change to the bottle, there is rarely any real necessity to do so. The majority of breastfeeding problems can be overcome with the right support and information. However, some problems are difficult to overcome – especially if they haven't been dealt with soon enough. And a few women just don't like breastfeeding even when it's going well on a physical level. If you decide that breastfeeding is not for you, that you're not enjoying it, or that it's become a struggle, do your best not to feel guilty (yes, easier said than done sometimes!). Regret is natural – many things in life don't turn out the way we would have hoped. But feeling guilty is a waste of energy, so try to feel good about your decision, feel positive about any breastfeeding you have done (however limited, your baby will have benefited), and then get on with enjoying your son or daughter!

Whatever your reasons, you'll need to know the simplest way to make the changeover. The same goes for WORKING if you've decided you can't/don't wish to try EXPRESSING BREAST MILK for those times when you're not around. The first rule is never to stop breastfeeding suddenly. A gradual run-down of your milk supply gets your body used to the lessening demands, and prevents any build-up of milk which could lead to ENGOR-GEMENT (and then BLOCKED DUCTS, and possibly a breast infection). Your baby may already be on some COMPLEMEN-TARY AND SUPPLEMENTARY BOTTLES after breastfeeds, which are, at least, a step in the direction of change. You can increase the amount of formula he's having by giving him an extra ounce or two at each 'top-up', and/or replacing a breastfeed with a bottle feed. Drop the breastfeeds gradually by substituting a bottle and leaving a few days between each separate change. If your baby has been fully breastfed, then the change should be along the same lines – a few days between each dropped breastfeed will give your body the chance to adjust. If you find yourself getting engorged, then gentle expressing, enough to simply soften the breast, will help.

Don't feel, by the way, that your baby must have a transition period on a bottle before he gets his drinks (or some of his drinks) from CUPS. Plenty of breastfed babies have never even seen a bottle, and from about six months or so start to take juice, water or milk in some sort of trainer cup. And returning to work rarely means complete WEANING from the breast unles that's what you want. One of the sadder aspects about making a change from breast to bottle, is, in my view, that too often it's a process that happens by itself – to the regret of the mother. If you've been topping-up with formula milk, or substituting formula for breast milk, because you feel you don't have enough milk, you can find your milk supply dwindles naturally without any conscious effort on your part. If you're keen to breastfeed, the use of formula in the early weeks should be the very last resort.

CHEESE*

Cheese is a good source of nutrients, especially calcium and protein. Introduce it in very small amounts at first, as the foreign protein in it may prove upsetting to the baby's digestion. I think that six months is a reasonable minimum age or later if there is ALLERGY in your family. Cheese is a fairly common allegen, so it's sensible to go cautiously at first.

First cheese can be cottage cheese, which is mild and soft-textured and you can mix it with pieces of fruit or vegetables. Buy those varieties of cottage cheese without salt in them if you can. Curd cheese is another good alternative. When your baby's about eight months old you can introduce other cheeses, though avoid strong flavours and the highly-spiced or highly-salted types. Gouda is a good one to try. If you want to avoid additives in your baby's food, read the labels on packaged cheese – many of them do have added colour. A small amount of cheese grated on top of a dish gives a nutritional bonus to a meal, and gives your baby a first chance to taste small amounts of it without it being the main part of the meal. Once you're happy your baby's ready for larger amounts of cheese, you can give a cube or a strip as finger food, or grate and chop some cheese for a baby old enough to have the co-ordination to pick up such small pieces.

When? From the second stage of WEANING for soft cheese (ie cottage or curd), then progressing to other cheeses.

CHEMICALS AND BREAST MILK

Every so often, concern is expressed about the effect of environmental chemicals on BREAST MILK. We live in a polluted world, and poisons can be breathed in (from the air), eaten (contaminated food) and even taken in via the skin (in the case of people who work with chemicals in industry). Certain toxins have been found to be stored in the body, and when the breast milk of women who have been exposed to high levels has been analysed, some experts have expressed anxiety about the safety of breastfed babies as a result. Currently, the World Health Organisation is pressing for action, and for more research. Calls for women to abandon breastfeeding because of this make little sense, however. The alternative is to give formula milk based on cow's milk. But environmental pollution may as easily affect cows, who have eaten grass near fields that may have been sprayed, or who may have had high doses of drugs or hormones or other elements in the formula, like vegetable oils for example, which may have been subject to chemical hazards in their plant form. The difference with breast milk is that you do have some measure of control over your own exposure to poisons. You may even be protecting your baby against the risks of exposure by giving him a healthy start in life. It is a scandal that not enough attention is paid to these problems, but to suggest that women bottle feed instead is alarmist and pointless.

CHERRIES*

Cherries can be eaten raw – you'll need to stone and chop them finely for a baby of course – or cooked. You may not need to sweeten them, but if they are too tart when cooked, add a little apple juice. Small amounts of cherries are nice mixed in with cottage cheese, yoghurt or other fruit. When you buy cherries for a baby, look for firm, shiny ones, as they will be at their best in this state.

When? From the second stage of WEANING.

CHEWING

Babies on solid food need to chew in order to encourage the production of saliva, which is the first stage of digestion. It's also good for jaw development. FINGER FOOD will encourage your baby to learn to chew, as opposed to suck, and this will extend his range of acceptable foods. Teeth are useful for chewing – but they aren't essential! Your baby will be able to bite and chew certain foods long before he has a mouthful of teeth, and in fact a baby's gums are quite hard, as you can feel if you ever put your finger in. Don't be frightened to offer lumps in your baby's food, even if he's still grinning gummily at a year. Plenty of babies have only one or two teeth at this age (and some have none), but they need to cope with food that's more than just mush.

CHICKEN*

Chicken is a versatile meat for babies and young children and it's usually quite popular. The best chicken to buy hasn't been intensively reared or force-fed. You usually have to buy it from a specialist poulterers although some of our larger supermarkets are selling it, alongside the 'normal' chicken. It's more expensive, but the improved flavour makes it worth the extra. Whatever chicken you end up getting, make sure it's defrosted before you cook it (whether it's intended for adults, children or babies). Partially defrosted chicken is thought to be responsible for numerous cases of food poisoning – and that's especially unpleasant, and dangerous, in a baby. And remember, don't give chicken with bones in it to a baby as smaller bones may break off and choke him. Otherwise, he can enjoy chicken in most of the ways you are likely to prepare it for the rest of the family, though avoid giving him chicken that is salted or spiced. He shouldn't have greasy, fried chicken, either, although fried chicken *without* a lot of fat remaining should be fine for a baby of over about eight months.

When? From the second stage of WEANING. Fried chicken from about eight months.

CHOCOLATE

Babies who have been slipped a piece of choccie by a doting relative who may not know or care about your feelings on sweet things, show their feelings of appreciation very clearly. But like sweets, cake and biscuits, the longer you can stave off chocolate, the better. There *is* a small amount of goodness in chocolate (there is iron in the cocoa powder, and milk in milk chocolate) –

47

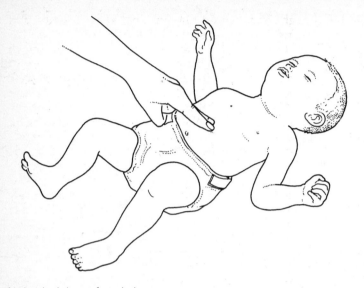

Abdominal thrust for a baby
Make sure that the infant is lying on a firm surface and that his head is tilted back to open the airway. Place the first two fingers of one hand on the upper abdomen, between the navel and the breastbone, and press inward and upward sharply. The thrust must be hard and sharp enough to dislodge the obstruction. This can be repeated up to four times.

and tiny amounts, occasionally, are nothing to become too distressed about. Chocolate is a well-known allergen, though, and in families with a history of food ALLERGY, or in a baby with suspected FOOD INTOLERANCE, it should be avoided completely for at least the first year. CAROB POWDER can be a substitute for chocolate in cooking.

CHOKING

All parents fear this happening to their babies and it is a real risk. Babies need someone with them at all times when they're eating, so prompt action can be taken if something 'goes down the wrong way'. It's possible to choke on breast milk although this isn't dangerous. If the baby splutters and comes off the breast,

48

hold him upright and comfort him and that's that. However, it can make feeding time unpleasant and there are ways to avoid it. It's more likely to happen when there's a fast flow of milk which overwhelms a new or newish baby; once he's reached the age of a couple of months or so he's usually able to deal with breast milk at whatever speed it comes. Until that stage is reached, it can help EXPRESSING BREAST MILK a little before you put the baby on, this sets off the LET-DOWN REFLEX so it's already working by the time your baby starts to suck and he doesn't get a fright.

Babies shouldn't be left with a bottle of milk propped up beside them so that they can feed themselves. 'Bottle propping' as it's known, can cause choking, or the baby can inhale regurgitated milk. In any case, a baby needs the comfort of being held securely while being fed, as well as the milk itself. (Bottle-propping may be the only way a bottle feeding mother of TWINS can cope on occasions, however; she should always watch over the one with the propped bottle, and make sure the twins take it in turns to be held while being fed.)

Babies are more likely to choke on foods they can't suck. Recent figures show that fatalities from choking in babies under six months have reduced considerably in the past few years. It's presumed that the main reason for this is the fact that solid food is being introduced at an older age than previously, and that babies of three months are far less likely to be given food they cannot cope with, and are likely to be still on milk alone. This is another good argument for delaying the introduction of solids (see WEANING). Always stay with your baby when he's eating, even if he can chew and swallow quite well. It's easy for him to break off a piece of food that's too big, and the horrifying thing about choking is the fact that the spluttering that accompanies it isn't loud like a cry, so you might not even hear it in the next room. At least if you're with your baby you can take prompt action if he starts to choke: get the piece of food out of his throat with your finger if you can reach it; if you can't, then turn him upside down and slap him on the back until he coughs it out or use the abdominal thrust. For older babies and toddlers who can stand, use the Heimlich Manoeuvre. Small objects of all sorts should be kept away from babies who are old enough to pick things up, in case they put them in their mouths. Remember that peanuts are especially dangerous to babies and young children and that if one is inhaled, the oil in the peanut can cause severe lung damage, even when the nut has been removed.

CITRUS FRUITS*

Grapefruits, lemons, limes, oranges are all famous for being rich in vitamin C. They have other valuable nutrients, too, such as potassium, and some of the B vitamins. Most babies will find the taste of the raw fruit too sharp, so you need to cook them, which will reduce the strength of the flavour.

When? From the second stage of WEANING.

CLEFT LIP AND/OR PALATE

A cleft lip and/or palate is an abnormality present at birth, but it is caused at some time in the first half of pregnancy by the failure of the upper lip and/or palate to fuse together. The condition leads to feeding difficulties; the lips may not be able to close on the nipple or teat as they would do normally, and in the case of a cleft palate, the milk may not be able to go directly down the throat, but instead exits down the nose. Skilled surgery means that the long-term problems of a child with this condition are very minor, and most babies born like this are able to feed normally by the end of the first year, even if there is further surgery to come. In the meantime, you need help and support. Breastfeeding can sometimes be attempted, it depends on the severity of the cleft or clefts, and exactly where they are. Your baby may have a feeding plate fitted which will close off the cleft in the palate. If breast-feeding isn't possible, you can try EXPRESSING BREAST MILK and feed by bottle – perhaps a bottle with a special teat made to cope with the problem. The protective properties of breast milk will be especially valuable to a baby who is going through surgery and hospital stays, where infection is always a risk. Bottle feeding by formula may need a special teat, too. In some cases, the baby may need to be fed milk on a spoon, or even by a tube. Spoonfeeding with solid food is a bit messy if your baby has a cleft palate, unless the feeding plate he has is very effective, or the palate has been successfully closed by surgery. He may still get bits of food running down his nose – and this could

irritate and distress him. The whole situation will get better, and confidence in this will help you through a difficult time.
See USEFUL ADDRESSES

COELIAC DISEASE

Coeliac disease is a relatively uncommon disorder of the metabolism. A baby with coeliac disease is unable to digest GLUTEN, the protein found in certain cereals. Symptoms are a failure to thrive, and bulky, light-coloured and offensive bowel motions. You will only notice symptoms when your baby starts on mixed feeding. There is no cure and the only treatment is a gluten-free diet. If you stick to the diet, your child will be just as healthy as anyone else. In coeliac disease, the lining of the intestine becomes damaged by the gluten and this interferes with the way other nutrients are digested. It's not known what causes coeliac disease, but breastfeeding helps prevent it, along with avoiding early solids, especially gluten-containing cereals.
See USEFUL ADDRESSES

COFFEE

Don't give your baby coffee to drink, or coffee-flavoured foods. His system is not developed enough to cope with the CAFFEINE, and he may be fractious and irritable as a result. If you are breastfeeding, your BREAST MILK may be affected if you drink a lot of coffee.

COLIC

Whatever colic is, it makes babies cry and parents despair. It's usually defined as some sort of abdominal pain, and it tends to affect younger babies – generally not from birth, but more typically after a couple of weeks or so, getting better towards the end of the third or fourth month. Is it air, or WIND, trapped in the lower intestine that causes it? Is it tummy pain caused by sensitivity to formula milk? Or to traces of food in the breast milk? Is it irritation caused by cigarette fumes? Is it a sign of being 'overfull' of milk? Is it just a baby's immature digestive system having a few difficulties, perhaps LACTOSE intolerance? All these explanations have been put forward, and backed up with formal research. There's another body of opinion that puts colic down to less physical factors, and which doesn't agree that there's necessarily any pain present. This body of opinion says the baby is reacting to the mother's own stress and lack of confidence; he's crying because he is picking up her tension, perhaps as she bustles round getting the evening meal ready (a lot of colic happens in the evenings). I don't want to deny that babies can feel genuine distress, but I do very much doubt that a baby can pick up his mother's tension night after night, when he is otherwise warm, well-cared for and fed. To me, this sounds another way of blaming the mother for everything, and of echoing the idea that all mothers are neurotic. Yes, we always feel guilty about our children, and wonder what we're doing wrong – but I don't think it's fair to blame mothers for colic. It's far more likely to be a result of something that's actually irritating the baby's tummy in some way. Colicky babies sometimes go on to be susceptible to FOOD INTOLERANCE or to suffer from ECZEMA or asthma.

Ways you could try to soothe your baby include: relactating if you are bottle feeding (see CHANGING: FROM BOTTLE TO BREAST); cutting out dairy products from your own diet (you need to do this for a week before you are likely to see any effects, and make sure you get sensible dietary advice if you need to do this long-term, to replace important missing nutrients); cutting out/down on tea, coffee, cola and other stimulants with CAF-FEINE in them which you take habitually; stopping SMOKING (or get your partner to do so); allowing your baby to feed from one breast per feed, if that's what he seems to want to do; allow him to feed on and off all evening, if that's what he seems to want; give him a dummy if you feel he is over-feeding, and yet needs some sucking comfort. In addition, you can help your baby calm down and cope better with his tummy pain by usual and unusual ways of settling him: a baby soother tape (available from record shops); soft music; cuddling and rhythmic rocking – side-to-side, up-and-down, whatever he likes best; carry him in a baby sling; suspend his carrycot from the ceiling in a special swinging hammock (you need to buy the proper thing – see USEFUL ADDRESSES); take him into a darkened, quiet room. Medication for colic is available from your doctor and over-the-counter at the chemists. I would be sceptical about these remedies, not just because I've met so few mothers who are convinced that they really and truly help, but also because one very widely prescribed remedy was withdrawn as it seemed to be linked with COT DEATH (though there's no proof it ever actually caused a cot death). So I think that we need to be very careful when giving drugs of any sort to a baby.

Colic does disappear in the first three to four months on the whole, and it's very rare for it to persist beyond the first six months. Do your best to get support and help if your baby is colicky. For instance, you need another person from time to time to cuddle and hold the baby for you, simply so you can feel you are a separate person again.

COLOSTRUM

Colostrum is the fluid produced in your breasts during pregnancy and in the first days after the birth. It's made in small quantities compared to breast milk but it's highly concentrated and very valuable nutritionally. It contains ANTIBODIES, and it's an excellent laxative. Some research has shown that even one feed of colostrum has significant benefits in raising the baby's immunity levels. So colostrum is both adequate and beneficial for your baby. Over a period of several days after the birth, the colostrum – creamy and yellowish – changes to breast milk, which is thinner and is white or even bluish in colour.

COLOURINGS

See ADDITIVES AND COLOURINGS

COMPLEMENTARY AND SUPPLEMENTARY BOTTLES

Complementary and supplementary bottles are bottles of FORMULA MILK given to a baby who's also breastfed. To define the terms more exactly, complementary bottles, or 'comps' or 'top-ups', are given after breastfeeding. Supplementary bottles are given instead of a breastfeed.

Not to beat about the bush, the introduction of bottles is one of the commonest reasons why breastfeeding fails. It is the *cause* of feeding problems, not the solution to them. If you want to continue breastfeeding, and you want you and your baby to decide when to stop, you will do your utmost to avoid bottles of formula milk. BREASTFEEDING responds to demand and you can only establish a milk supply if you stimulate it by putting your baby to the breast and allowing him to feed as much and as often as he wants. This means frequent, unscheduled feeding, especially at first. Bottles upset this 'demand and supply' mechanism, simply by reducing the demand made on the supply. Top-ups, or supplementary feeds, are often introduced because the mother fears her supply of breast milk is inadequate. Let's see what happens when this is done. We'll take a situation where your baby is not gaining weight as she should. You introduce formula milk one evening after a breastfeed and your baby has perhaps a four ounce top-up – and then what? Your baby may drop off to sleep on a full tummy; he may sleep longer than normal, and wake up later for a breastfeed. Your breast milk supply will be stimulated less, and the problem of insufficient milk (if that's what it was) becomes greater. Or you may feel your milk supply is adequate for a reasonably satisfactory weight gain, but your baby continues to cry after some or all feeds and you feel your milk isn't satisfying him. If you give him top-ups, he settles better. But you may find that the top-ups reduce your milk supply in the same way and that your milk ceases to satisfy your baby simply because there isn't enough of it.

Of course, I'm not saying that the problem of insufficient milk is an imaginary one, or that babies who are otherwise thriving are always fully satisfied on breast milk at every feed. Far from it. These situations are real and distressing – all mothers react to the sound of their babies cries and it's not at all surprising that they seek a solution to it. Nor am I saying that your milk supply will disappear as soon as you give one feed of formula milk. But if your breastfed baby seems to be crying for more milk, then give him more – from the breast. He may even need waking up in the day in order to feed more frequently, and therefore build up your supply to one that will keep him growing as he should. More rest for you and attention to your diet will help as well (see DIET AND BREASTFEEDING). Ask someone who knows about breastfeeding to check your baby's well positioned at the breast, as poor fixing can lead to inadequate feeding (see POSITION AT BREAST). After a few days, your milk supply will catch up with your baby's needs and you can probably stop the extra feeds. But changing back to the breast is difficult after bottlefeeds have caused a dwindling of your milk supply, and it is not always possible (see CHANGING: FROM BREAST TO BOTTLE).

It should be said that some breastfed babies don't like formula milk, or bottles, and sick the whole lot up again, or just don't manage to work the teat. Even babies who take the bottle may not even be hungry – they may just suck on the teat because, like Everest, it's there! 'Sucky' babies will suck on anything for the sheer pleasure of it. So, you run the risk of turning your baby to bottle-sucking instead of breastfeeding, too. The techniques are different, and a baby who gets used to the bottle teat can find it hard to switch back to the breast. She may start to fight at the breast, irritated that the milk isn't coming in the same way and at the same rate as when she sucks at the bottle (see BREAST REFUSAL). The different way you hold her when breastfeeding, close to you and facing you, may irritate her too. This problem doesn't seem to arise very frequently with babies who are given only the occasional bottle, whether of juice, formula or expressed breast milk but this is an impression of mine and I've seen no research to prove it. It does suggest to me however, that babies remain adaptable until bottles become more regular, and this is reassuring for mothers who have to give a bottle of something (EXPRESSING BREAST MILK is obviously preferable) on occasions. I do think the confusion between nipple and teat is more likely to arise if the mother is also suffering from a dwindling milk supply, which may make her baby more likely to prefer the bottle.

There's also the important aspect of FOOD INTOLERANCE. Even one small formula feed may disrupt the mechanism that protects your baby against ALLERGY – exclusive breastfeeding is the best protection. Is it worth the risk? CRYING can be hard to cope with, and so can COLIC. But a feed of formula milk only offers a short-term solution, if it offers any solution at all, and the price you pay for the possibility of an hour or so's peace can be high. In my view, the practice of having a can of formula and a bottle and a teat in your cupboard 'just in case' when you're breastfeeding has nothing to recommend it at all. You're quite likely to use it when you're longing to sleep at one in the morning and all your baby does is feed and/or cry.

Is there ever any case for using bottles with a breastfed baby? In a very few cases, a baby who fails to thrive on breast milk may actually need formula milk, because despite everything the mother does, she cannot build up a supply. In some countries, a MILK BANK exists for this situation, and if we were less queasy about WET-NURSING in this country we'd accept that this was a possible way out, too. But given that neither of those options is likely to be available, then formula of some sort is advisable. It sometimes happens that the mother has, in fact, loads of milk, but the baby still doesn't grow well. This problem needs investigating, in case the baby has a growth disorder or metabolic deficiency. Putting the baby on formula milk rarely solves this problem, and may set up allergies that breastfeeding could have prevented. If formula milk has to be used, it's best kept to a minimum and offered after the breastfeed so the breasts get maximum stimulation. For a mother who cannot build up her supply sufficiently well to fully breastfeed her baby, this may be the best compromise, and the only way she can continue to breastfeed at all. It *is* sometimes possible to get this sort of combined feeding down to a fine art, maintaining a breast milk supply for weeks or even months and keeping a check on the amount of formula used. More often, though, the breast milk supply does trail away.

The situation of a working mother is quite a bit different again. In most cases, the baby is already several months old, and when this is so, your breast milk is far less likely to dwindle away to nothing because of bottles, and older babies usually seem clever enough to cope with both sucking techniques, especially with a mother whose milk supply is maintained (see WORKING).

Of course, bottles don't have to be filled with formula milk. Some mothers feel they always have a less abundant milk supply in the evenings and so they express milk in the mornings when they have more, and supply the shortfall in a bottle. This has the double advantage of keeping the baby off formula milk and maintaining the milk supply.

CONSTIPATION

Constipation is the difficulty of passing stools because they are generally dry so the baby needs to strain to push them out, and this can be painful. Bowel motions are usually infrequent, but don't mistake the long gaps that breastfed babies sometimes have between bowel motions, as a sign of constipation so long as these are soft and easily passed. Exclusively breastfed babies are never constipated. But breastfed babies taking anything other than breast milk, are sometimes, and so are bottle fed ones. Extra fluids in the diet can help a great deal, and a few spoonfuls of good old-fashioned prune juice is an effective and safe remedy, as well. Some babies get constipated as a result of a certain food their digestive system has yet to cope with efficiently, so it's worth thinking along these lines if your baby suffers during the earlier stages of WEANING (eggs are a common culprit, for instance). Frequent and/or uncomfortable constipation in a baby needs discussing with your health visitor or doctor.

CONTRACEPTION

During the time you are fully breastfeeding, you are less likely to ovulate (release an egg), and therefore less likely to become pregnant. This is because the hormone PROLACTIN which produces the milk, also prevents ovulation, and therefore menstruation. This all sounds pretty good in theory, and if you're interested in natural forms of contraception, or 'child-spacing' as it's known sometimes, then breastfeeding exclusively for at least six months and thereafter partially for a further year or more, is likely to delay your fertility considerably. Exactly how long varies from woman to woman. Some women find that their periods return as soon as their baby starts spacing out his feeds. Others find that even one short feed a day keeps them from menstruating and that things only get back to normal when breastfeeding ceases entirely. And there are lots of variations in between these two extremes. If you are keen to avoid pregnancy, and you wish, like most women, to carry on having intercourse, then you cannot rely on breastfeeding acting as a guaranteed contraceptive. For one thing, it's rarely possible to know when you've ovulated (though you can learn to 'read' your own vaginal secretions, which change at ovulation), and menstruation happens a fortnight *after* you've ovulated. It's therefore possible to become pregnant without having had a period at all between your babies.

So, if you want to use artificial contraception, then what are you going to do? This isn't the book to assess all the various methods available to you, but if you're thinking of the Pill, you will want to know if it affects breastfeeding. Current family planning practice is to avoid prescribing the combined Pill – the one that has the hormone oestrogen and progesterone. This has been shown to reduce the quantity of breast milk produced, so obviously it's to be avoided. The usual alternative is the pro-gestogen-only Pill, sometimes known as the POP or the mini-Pill, which contains only one (artificial) hormone, and is not thought to have any effect on lactation, or on the baby. However, there's no real proof of this, and minute amounts of hormone do reach the breast milk, and therefore the baby. Is this harmful? It's just not known. One expert states that the amount of hormone received by a breastfed baby from his POP-taking mum over a period of two years, is equivalent to just one tablet. He compares it to SMOKING, which he says is far more potentially harmful to the baby.

I do think we still have a lot to learn about long-term effects of hormonal contraceptives, and the effect on breastfed babies is just one of the aspects that cannot yet be proved to be safe or harmful. If you want to avoid all the theoretical or real risks to yourself or your baby, you'll think of some other method. It's up to you to discuss it with your doctor, or family planning clinic. You may decide that a good, effective convenient contraceptive is worth the small cloud of doubt that accompanies it. One thing you should bear in mind is that the POP needs to be taken at the same time every day. If motherhood makes you forgetful, or you find it hard to stick to routines at this time, then maybe this in itself should make you think of another method.

CONVENIENCE FOODS

This generally means foods that have been commercially pre-pared, in order to save on cooking time. The healthiest diet, for babies and anyone else, is made up of fresh ingredients – but we live in the real world where we have to cope with other pressures on our time and energy, and convenience foods aren't necessarily unhealthy. So get into the way of reading labels, and avoid foods with ADDITIVES AND COLOURINGS, or added

SUGAR. Avoid foods for babies with added SALT, too. Salt-free convenience-foods are less easy to find because salt acts as a preservative. BABY FOODS are usually more suitable for a baby or toddler than other sorts of convenience foods, as they have been specially-prepared without additives, without salt and often without added sugar. Other convenience foods you could give to your baby, once he's well-established on solids, might include canned beans or pulses, canned vegetables, canned fruit (not the sort in syrup), and the same items frozen. Things like meat pies, pizzas, fish fingers and fish cakes almost always contain salt, and sometimes colouring and preservatives, and so they are best avoided.
See also FROZEN FOODS

CORNFLOUR

Cornflour may be used as a thickener in baby foods and other convenience foods. There's very little nutritional value in it, but as it's used in very small quantities it's unlikely to take the place of other more valuable foods.

COT DEATH

Tragically, about one baby in every 500 dies suddenly without any apparent cause or previous serious illness. The death is called a 'cot death' as many of its victims die in their cots or their prams, seemingly in their sleep. The other term is SIDS, or 'Sudden Infant Death Syndrome'.

Various theories attempt to explain cot death. It may be a mystery virus; it could be some sort of devastating allergic response; it could be some previously unsuspected breathing disorder. We just don't know. However, one thing is clear: breastfeeding offers some protection. Cot death is less common in babies who are exclusively breastfed at the time they die. Is there something vital in breast milk which defeats a virus which causes cot death? Or is it something to do with the way breastfed babies may be more likely to sleep close to their mothers or anyway have more physical contact with their mothers, so slight signs of illness or breathing disturbance are spotted straight away? Whatever the reason, it seems important to encourage

59

and support breastfeeding for the first six months (when cot death is most common) as a preventative measure. This is especially important for mothers who have had a previous child which has died in this way, because we know that a new baby in the family who have already experienced a cot death is actually at greater risk than a baby in a family with no such history.
See USEFUL ADDRESSES

COTTAGE CHEESE

See CHEESE

COURGETTE*

Cook courgettes in the minimum of water, or else steam or sauté them. They're a good starter vegetable for young babies, as they can be mashed if necessary, and the flavour isn't too strong. Cooked slices, cubes or sticks of courgette make finger food for older babies.

When? From the second stage of WEANING.

COW'S MILK

Great for baby cows – not so great for baby humans. Most FORMULA MILK is based on cow's milk, and of course the ordinary full-fat pasteurised milk that we have in the UK is as well. When we talk about milk, this is what we mean – and in this entry, this is what I'm referring to as well. In Western cultures, we tend to drink a lot of milk although this isn't the case in other countries of the world. Milk's a highly nutritious food – it contains protein, vitamins (mainly A and D), minerals (such as calcium) and fats. And because it comes to us ready to drink, and (in the UK) it's sometimes actually delivered to the house, it's also highly convenient. But it isn't essential. Plenty of perfectly healthy people never drink milk beyond infancy. All the components of milk are available in other foods, so a child who never drinks cow's milk doesn't have to be at a disadvantage nutritionally speaking. However, because of the way we base so much of our food intake on cows' milk, it can be difficult to avoid it, and substituting other food and drink needs thought and organisation.

Cow's milk intolerance is actually more common than we used to think. Some people are allergic to the protein in cow's milk; others may not produce lactase, the enzyme that aids the digestion of LACTOSE, the sugar present in milk. Either way, symptoms of ALLERGY in a baby or child can vary from stomach pains, failure to thrive, skin and respiratory disorders, constant vomiting and/or diarrhoea, to less obviously physical signs like unsettled and/or distressed behaviour and sleeplessness (see also FOOD INTOLERANCE). The best way of avoiding cow's milk intolerance in your baby is to breastfeed exclusively for the first six months, and to introduce cow's milk very gradually thereafter. This allows your baby's system to build up a resistance to the foreign protein in the milk. If and when you do give your baby cow's milk, boil it and dilute it half and half with water until the age of about nine months. This is a precautionary measure as the boiling breaks down the protein, and the diluting reduces its strength. Of course, both processes also reduce its nutritive value, so it would be very unwise for boiled, diluted milk to form a major part of your baby's diet. It's fine for most babies as an occasional drink, or for mixing with other foods. The rest of your baby's milk should ideally be breast milk, or failing that, formula milk. Most babies, by the age of a year, can tolerate ordinary pasteurised milk without boiling and diluting.

Skimmed and semi-skimmed milk This usually refers to cow's milk that has had the fat content removed in the processing. Skimmed milk has had all the fat taken away; semi-skimmed milk has had half the fat taken away. Along with the fat – and the calories in it – go the fat-soluble vitamins A and D. Once babies are on milks other than breast milk or formula milk, they should be given whole milk only – not skimmed or semi-skimmed. This is because they need the fat and the VITAMINS to stay healthy. UK government recommendations state that whole milk is the best milk for all children up to the age of five, though semi-skimmed milk is permissable from the age of two for a child on a good mixed diet. This isn't to say that skimmed or semi-skimmed is actively harmful. But in this country where we drink a lot of milk and give even more to our children, a baby is likely to get much of his daily food intake in the form of milk. This is why it should be whole milk, as anything less would mean he could be missing out. On the other hand, if he's given the occasional drink of skimmed or semi-skimmed milk, or if skimmed or semi-skimmed milk forms part of another dish, and it's not actually substituting his usual formula, breast or ordinary full-fat pasteurised milk, he won't be harmed. Remember that the best milk for all babies in their first year is breast milk, or in its absence formula milk, and that babies who are intolerant to cow's milk will be intolerant to skimmed or semi-skimmed milk, too.

CRACKED AND SORE NIPPLES

See NIPPLES

CREAM

If your baby is already on cow's milk (ordinary full-fat pasteurised milk rather than formula), and he's coping, then a small amount of cream very occasionally will be tolerated, though remember it's a 'rich', that is, very fatty, food, and too much will overload a baby's tummy and be hard to digest. Cream should be never more than an occasional part of a healthy diet for anyone because of its high fat content.

When? From about nine months, or after your baby has shown he can tolerate whole cow's milk.

CRISPS

Crisps aren't normally suitable for babies in the age range which concerns this book. Most varieties are high in salt, and many are artificially flavoured. They are too hard and, well, *crispy*, for a baby to chew sufficiently well, even if she has teeth at the front and back.

CRYING

Babies cry – all of them, at some time. It's their only way of indicating hunger or distress. Crying can be a serious problem in itself and it's very hard for parents to cope at times. This isn't the book to explore the whole phenomenon, and you should look elsewhere for a full discussion, but here I'll deal with the ways in which crying can relate to food and feeding (see BOOKLIST). In the first weeks feed your baby when he cries, if you are breastfeeding. The chances are he'll settle because he needed to feed to take away his hunger pangs. Frequent feeding, is the best way to establish a reliably adequate milk supply anyway. Bottle fed babies usually need feeding less often than breastfed ones, and they may cry because of thirst (see FORMULA MILK). If you have recently fed your baby with a bottle of formula milk, then try a small amount of water if he cries (with breast milk there's no problem in sorting out the difference as it supplies all your baby's fluid needs as well, so putting him to the breast is fine). But if the baby is constantly crying despite frequent feeding, it may be organic in origin – in other words, your baby may be suffering from illness. It's important to have your doctor's opinion, even if, or especially if, he manages to reassure you that there's nothing seriously wrong.

Other food related causes of crying in the early months are WIND, COLIC and ALLERGY or FOOD INTOLERANCE. The latter can show up as frequent crying in a bottle fed baby who has an intolerance to COW'S MILK. Breastfed babies sometimes react to substances in their mother's milk (see DIET AND BREASTFEEDING). Food intolerance can manifest itself as crying in a previously contented baby, for example. A normally breastfed baby may cry after being given a bottle of formula milk – maybe it's giving him a pain. Or your baby may react to a food he's never had before by crying.

If your baby is underweight he may cry a lot because he is often hungry but check his health to make sure this is the reason. Babies and toddlers still cry with hunger as they get older – they don't have the language or the understanding to pinpoint and then communicate the problem. It's a good idea to have some healthy snacks on hand once your baby's on mixed feeding and they will help keep her quiet while you get her meal ready.

CUPS

The first cup for a baby should be a 'training beaker' – it has a lid with a spout. With this, she can adapt her established sucking technique and draw the liquid up through the spout. Ordinary cups can be used too, but babies aren't good at slurping and swallowing, which is what they have to do at first, until at least towards the end of the first year. The spouted cup reduces the risk of spills, too, as the child can lift it and use it without tipping the fluid out and it encourages her to be independent. (Of course, babies soon learn they can make an entertaining shower of droplets by turning the cup upside down and shaking it . . . a skill to be discouraged.)

There are many different sorts of cups available. At first, one without a handle seems easier and lighter to hold. Handled cups should have a handle on each side, which makes balancing the cup easier. You can buy weighted cups which are less likely to tip (only important anyway when the lid is removed) but for a baby under a year these are too heavy. I prefer transparent cups, as you can see straight away what and how much your baby's drinking, although that's not a vital point. Babies themselves probably prefer bright colours and pictures. A cup with an interchangable travel lid, that keeps the cup completely closed, is useful. Alternatively, you can buy cups with a sort of double top, where a turn of the lid closes off the spout in the manner of a Parmesan cheese container. Cleaning spouted cups is a bore, rinsing isn't enough and neither is dishwashing, especially if your baby uses his to drink milk out of. The debris collects round the holes and inside the spout itself, and you need to give it a good poke round with something like a dead matchstick and a scrub with a BOTTLE BRUSH. For babies under a year who regularly drink milk from a spouted cup, the occasional steep in STERILISING solution after a good clean will prevent bugs developing.

Changing to cups   Babies aren't usually able to manage a cup until they're at least five months old – and they're not especially proficient at getting much out for at least another month or two. A spouted cup, sometimes called a 'trainer cup', is best to start with, though you can hold a normal cup up to a baby's lips for him to slurp. But the spout allows your baby to use a sucking technique to draw the milk up, and of course there's less risk of spills.

Most babies are having fluids other than breast milk by the end of the first year, though breast milk is a nutritious drink for all ages. Babies on formula milk may drink water or juice as well as milk from early on. In both cases, cup-drinking can be seen as a useful skill, rather than as essential, some bottles (of juice or water) or breast milk could supply all the drinks a baby would need for the whole of the first year. A good time to think about introducing a cup is when your baby is becoming established on solid food. Offer a cup at mealtimes, in place of a breast or bottle feed if you're thinking about cutting down on breast or bottle. You'll need to put it to your baby's mouth at first, but as time goes on he'll get the hang of it and pick it up himself. It's an idea to deliberately repeat the word 'cup' or 'drink' as you give him it, and as you see him use it – this will help him to learn the word so he can indicate when he's thirsty.

Gradually increasing your baby's use of the cup, by introducing it at every meal and offering a drink mid-morning and afternoon, will probably mean he'll get most of his fluid from it by the time he's a year old, unless you maintain breast or bottle feeds as well, which of course many mothers do. Don't worry if your baby doesn't seem to enjoy a cup, and rejects it in favour of breast or bottle. This won't last for ever – in fact, it's unusual beyond 12 months – if you simply keep offering small drinks in the cup at every meal. Leave the cup on the tray for him and casually draw his attention to it from time to time, but don't insist on it by continually putting it to his mouth yourself or you will put him off even more.

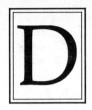

DAIRY PRODUCTS

This generic term includes all foods made from milk, and by extension, foods containing milk. Because of the milk content, children who are intolerant of COW'S MILK may have to avoid all dairy products – though this isn't necessarily the case. Small quantities may be acceptable, and food items such as YOGHURT or CHEESE which have the milk content modified by the benign bacteria, may be too. On the other hand, a child affected by cow's milk intolerance may also react to other foods, including other dairy products, because of its other constituents . . . and a child able to 'take' milk may react to other dairy products. Some children develop the ability to tolerate dairy products as they grow older, though such foods remain one of the prime 'suspect areas' in cases of FOOD INTOLERANCE.

DEHYDRATION

I have included dehydration, along with DIARRHOEA, because they are so closely connected with food and fluid intake, and so deserve entries. A severe loss of fluid from the body causes dehydration – and in an infant it's a potentially serious condition. It can be caused by fever and/or severe diarrhoea and VOMITING, which can devastatingly deplete the body of the essential fluids and salts it needs. You need to get immediate medical attention if your baby seems dehydrated. Signs of dehydration are obvious listlessness and 'floppiness', a sunken fontanelle (the soft spot on the top of the skull), and/or a lack of wet nappies despite the diarrhoea. If you think your baby may be dehydrated, then continue to breastfeed as often as the baby will take it. A bottle fed baby needs WATER or other clear fluids and *not* extra milk feeds, unless they are diluted half-and-half with water.

Babies whose diet includes solids should revert to fluids, either breast milk, clear fluids or half-strength milk feeds. You should have sachets of oral rehydration solution in the home – they're available from any chemist. Mix one according to directions and give it to your child.

DEMAND FEEDING

This phrase is used in contrast to SCHEDULED FEEDING, and it usually refers to BREASTFEEDING. We know that the breast milk supply responds best to frequent stimulation at first – that's the way the production line is established. We also know that you make as much milk as your baby needs if you allow him to feed when he wants to. As a result, the supply builds up to meet the demand if it's allowed to. It's on this principle that mothers can feed TWINS, or even more babies, as her milk supply gets correspondingly more stimulation. Demand feeding certainly makes sense. Hospitals used to insist on routine feeding – a feed every four hours, 10 minutes a side, and not at night – and this can spell disaster for breastfeeding. Few women can produce enough milk for their babies in these conditions. Even now, mothers still end up bottle feeding because many places only pay lip service to the idea of demand feeding and some midwives, health visitors and doctors may also still undermine breastfeeding by resisting the idea of demand feeding – old habits die hard. The irony is that it is scheduled feeding that is, in fact, modern, and mainly based on what was advised for babies fed unmodified cow's milk with a bottle (aided and abetted, of course, by the idea that babies were untamed monsters who needed regulating, that medical men knew better than mothers who needed to be regulated, too). Demand feeding doesn't mean you're bound to end up with a spoilt toddler who 'demands' everything at once. In fact, I prefer the term 'unrestricted feeding', invented by the Stanways, as it sounds a whole lot better (see BOOKLIST). You'll end up with a good milk supply, and a baby who has his pains of hunger satisfied – and that's a good start in life, surely!

How long should you feed on demand in this way? And what does it mean in practical terms? Do you have to be there, with your baby plugged in, 24 hours a day if necessary? In the first days after the birth, many babies only want occasional short feeds (though there are others who suck a lot right from the start). Then, you will probably notice that your baby starts to feed more frequently – nine to 12 feeds a day isn't unusual. Of course, it's sometimes difficult to say what constitutes a breast-feed as some feeds may be no more than apparently token sucks that get your baby off to sleep, and others may last quite a long time (an hour or more is normal, although some of this time is taken up with stopping and starting, winding, changing the baby, allowing her to rest between bouts of feeding, and so on). A SLEEPY BABY may need to be woken, in order to encourage him to make demands on your milk supply and get it underway.

Sometime in the first couple of months your baby will start to space his feeds out. This happens partly as a result of your breast milk supply becoming efficiently established, and partly as a result of the way your baby grows, taking more milk at each feed and becoming more efficient at doing so. A three-to-four hourly pattern is fairly typical, though this is unlikely to divide itself up absolutely regularly. Many babies, for example, go longer between morning feeds, and they tend to be shorter, building up to more frequent feeds in the evening, which tend to be long and lingering. So the image of the baby constantly at the breast is not a very typical one, although most babies have odd days or groups of days when this seems to be the only thing that will settle them. Once the breast milk supply is established, few mothers need to feed round the clock. Their babies thrive on six to eight feeds a day, most days. I should add that, when breastfeeding's going well, you don't actually count the feeds, and nor do you watch the clock to monitor its frequency, or to time the length of the feeds. It just happens.

Demand feeding can work two ways, as well. Babies who are healthy, thriving and growing well, can be encouraged to adopt a routine, once the milk supply's well-established. This means you can feed before you go out somewhere with your baby, in order to avoid having to feed him somewhere inconvenient. Wake him up just as you go to bed if it helps avoid being woken up by his hunger cries an hour later. If you're in the middle of your dinner, hand him to someone else to cuddle and distract for a short time until you finish . . . and so on. Mothers of older children who have to be taken to and from nursery or school often have to modify demand feeding in this way. It doesn't always work and you end up feeding when you don't want to, or where it isn't especially ideal. Or else your baby screams with hunger while you dash back home, pushing the pram through the driving rain – despite the sure-fire (you thought) tummy filler of a feed you gave him two hours before.

What about demand feeding for bottle fed babies? The usual practice in hospital is to encourage a sort of demand feeding, rather than to insist on the baby getting his regulation number of ounces at each feed, every so many hours. BOTTLE FEEDING mothers report that their babies do reach a routine in a few weeks (probably sooner than breastfed babies), and this is mainly because the baby is offered a constant amount of unchanging formula milk at each feed, which encourages regularity. There's no real reason to insist that demand feeding is the only way for bottle feeding, yet you'll want to be responsive to your baby's appetite and sensitive to his needs, rather than slavishly following a rigid pattern.

DESSERTS*

Keep desserts free from sugar and remember that babies don't have to have one after every lunch or tea. Try a slice or two of fruit, a milk pudding, or fresh fruit jellies ... there are lots of ideas. Bought desserts in baby food ranges do tend to be very sweet, but there are some perfectly acceptable varieties. Again, label-reading is the key. Avoid the packets of instant pud you whip up with milk – full of additives and colourings, sugar and fat – everyone's best off without these sorts of convenience foods.

DIARRHOEA

Diarrhoea is the frequent passage of loose stools, caused by the body's reaction to a stomach or digestive infection, or to other fever or illness. Don't confuse diarrhoea with the normal, loose, bright yellow stools of a fully-breastfed baby (which are often frequent as well). Diarrhoea in a breastfed baby is rarer than in a bottle fed baby, but it does occur, and can be identified as liquid, mucousy stools, possibly foul-smelling. Many babies get the odd touch of diarrhoea, and if your baby is otherwise healthy, drinking and eating normally, then there is nothing to worry about. The occasional green stool in a breastfed baby, or mucousy, loose stool in a bottle fed baby or one on mixed feeding, may look alarming but it's no cause for anxiety at all. Only if the diarrhoea persists over a period without getting better, or if your child shows other symptoms such as fever or vomiting, do you need to take any action. Contact your doctor or health visitor, and they'll advise you on the seriousness of the problem.

Maintain your child's fluid intake throughout his bout of diarrhoea, and give oral rehydration salts if the diarrhoea doesn't seem to be getting better by itself (see DEHYDRATION). Bottle fed babies may sometimes be better off on half-strength feeds – though see your doctor before you do this yourself. Breastfed babies simply need their usual breast milk, which will help them fight infection and cannot possible be 'too strong' for them to digest. A baby already on solids may want to revert to more breastfeeding when he's suffering from diarrhoea – that's fine, and beneficial to him.

If your baby's moving on to solids and he has diarrhoea it could just be a reaction to something he's eaten for the first time. Frequent diarrhoea, whether or not it's accompanied by any other obvious symptoms, needs to be discussed with your doctor. It could be a symptom of FOOD INTOLERANCE towards something or several things. Frequent diarrhoea is associated with failure to thrive and some metabolic disorders and severe food intolerance. Some bottle fed babies have diarrhoea that's caused by a sensitivity to cow's milk formula. Don't diagnose any of this yourself though – seek medical advice.

DIET

A good diet for a child in the first year will go from exclusive milk feeding in the first four to six months, to include a wide range of solid foods, taken at two or three meals a day, and supplemented with milk. The best milk for your baby throughout this time is BREAST MILK and other MILK should be introduced gradually, if at all, after six months. It's not helpful to real-life parents to state exact figures of how many grams of protein, carbohydrate and so forth your baby needs at any particular age. Babies are so very different from one another in this age group and you can't possibly organise your baby's intake in this way. It's far better to be guided by what you perceive your baby's needs to be, together with your own common sense, when you're deciding which foods and how much of them you should give your baby. If, by 12 months your baby's growing well and developing normally, if she enjoys most mealtimes, if her intake includes a minimum of sweet foods and she is continuing to increase her range of fresh (not packaged) solid foods, and getting used to different textures, then you are doing fine. As a rough guideline, a baby of this age needs some fruit or vegetables, some potato, bread or cereal, some meat, beans, fish, cheese or egg at most meals, supplemented with milk in some form.

See also WEANING

DIET AND BREASTFEEDING

Stick to sensible, healthy eating yourself when you're breastfeeding. There has been little research to prove that the quality of your breast milk plummets when you're not eating well, but the quantity may decrease. Women in developing countries manage to breastfeed, even when they are undernourished themselves and it's been found that the quality of breast milk is only seriously affected when the mother's diet is severely lacking in protein. That's hardly likely to happen in a Western country – our diets may be less than ideal in many ways, but a shortage of protein is not a problem. You can be sure your breast milk is the best possible food and drink for your baby. It is those women who aren't getting enough to eat themselves who find it more difficult to maintain the right quantity of milk for their babies. This may be one of the main reasons why mothers in poorer countries, who get barely enough to eat, may have to feed their babies a lot more frequently and for a lot longer, than we do in the West. Their breast milk supply needs stimulating much more often in order to maintain adequate production. But mothers in relatively affluent societies may not necessarily eat sufficiently well. It's easy to skip meals and forget about your own needs when you're caring for a new baby. However, if you want to increase your milk supply, think about eating better. Choose nourishing snacks instead of biscuits or cakes when you feel a bit peckish. Respond to your body's needs – if you feel hungry, and a lot of women do in the first weeks of breastfeeding, have some bread and cheese. Try to eat three times a day – it doesn't have to be a cooked meal as long as it keeps you well-fuelled. Try to avoid worrying about weight loss in the early weeks – formal weight-reduction diets aren't advisable at this stage.

There has not been a lot of work to show precisely what effects different sorts of diets have on the 'ingredients' of breast milk. Traces of foods do get through to the milk in some form and mothers report that their babies react to different foods. In most cases, the effects of these aren't very serious, and they are only temporary. You have a plateful of brussels sprouts for dinner one evening, and your baby seems a bit windy the next day. Or else you have a very spicy chilli con carne and you notice that your baby seems to have mild tummy pains. I have heard of many different foods having an effect on babies and you can't tell in advance what will or won't affect yours. So avoiding something simply because you're breastfeeding makes no sense at all, until, you notice that something does make a difference.

The question of FOOD INTOLERANCE is another matter. The newest work on ALLERGY indicates that some breastfed babies may have been sensitised to cow's milk protein in the uterus (because traces of it reach him via the bloodstream), for instance, and react to minute traces of cow's milk in the breast milk afterwards. The tiny traces present in the breast milk itself do not seem enough to precipitate sensitisation themselves, but if a baby has a drink of formula milk, this could be enough to lead to a reaction next time. If your breastfed baby suffers from COLIC or sleeplessness and shows any of the other symptoms of intolerance, it can be worth cutting out food items from your diet. CAFFEINE is one thing to start with, if you drink a great deal of tea, coffee or cola. Think about other items that could be causing a reaction, too. Babies with colic do sometimes improve if the mother cuts down on milk, and sometimes all dairy products too. If you do this for more than a few days, however, you'll need careful thought about replacing missing nutrients in your diet. Get advice from a diet-minded doctor, or else a dietician if you need to.

DIGESTIVE SYSTEM

Although the order in which digestion takes place is the same however a baby is fed, details of the process differ according to whether the baby is breast or bottle fed or receiving any solid food. If we talk about something being easier to digest than something else, we mean its components are metabolised more quickly (broken down and converted in order for the body to use them). Breast milk is easy to digest, for example, and this is one of the reasons why a breastfed baby will need more frequent feeding, generally speaking, than a bottle fed baby on formula milk – the stomach empties that much sooner, leaving the 'empty feeling' which leads to hunger. In a baby, disorders of the digestive system are potentially serious, because they mean he can't extract the right nourishment from his food. Examples of disorders that have this effect include PKU (phenylketonuria), COELIAC DISEASE, FOOD INTOLERANCE and disorders such as diabetes, which prevent the body from manufacturing the right substances to aid digestion. Other, usually temporary, illnesses, such as GASTROENTERITIS are caused by infections of the digestive tract. Obviously, temporary illness like this needs medical treatment if it persists.

DRIED FOODS*

Many BABY FOODS are presented as dried foods, for example baby FORMULA MILK is usually sold direct to mothers as a dried product. Solid foods intended for babies are available in dried form, and you usually have to reconstitute with water (boiled and cooled for the younger baby) or sometimes with made-up formula milk or expressed breast milk (see EXPRESSING BREAST MILK). There's nothing really wrong with them, and they're certainly very handy as an instant meal, especially as you only need to use a tiny amount at a time if that's all you need. However, you do need to read the labels if you want to avoid something like sugar (often present, either as sucrose or some other sugar like glucose or dextrose), or COW'S MILK (many varieties have skimmed milk powder in them). They tend to be very smooth and babies who get too used to them get rather conservative about 'real' food.

Dried fruits are rather different. You can soak dried pieces of fruit for purées and juices, or as a basis for other dishes. A piece of dried apricot, for example, makes a good, long-lasting, chewy finger food for an older baby able to cope with it. I've found that slices of dried fruits – dried bananas, pears, apples and other examples are a useful snack to offer on a shopping trip but you need to brush your child's teeth afterwards, as they are sweet and sticky. You can get a wide variety at wholefood shops and some supermarkets. Choose the sort without added mineral oil (put in as a preservative) or else wash thoroughly before giving them to your baby.

DRINKS

Breastfed babies under four to six months don't need anything else apart from breast milk. Normal, healthy, full-term breastfed babies are still routinely offered water or sugar water (dextrose or glucose solution) in hospital. There is no justification for this and it works against breastfeeding as the baby is less inclined to suck. Bottlefed babies on formula milk may need water (boiled and cooled) in hot weather, when they are ill or just in order to satisfy their thirst. Fruit juices, or the new herbal juices, are no longer considered essential, and breastfeeding mothers might even find it difficult to get their babies to drink them because of both the taste and the new experience of bottle and teat. They too may damage the milk supply, and they may activate FOOD INTOLERANCE in some babies. If your baby seems thirsty, give him breast milk or water depending on how you are feeding – it's much simpler!

Later on, at the 4–6 month stage, offer your baby other drinks – vegetable and fruit juices (unsweetened and diluted), cow's milk or water – as part of his 'taste education' and as part of every meal. He may also want a drink at several other points during the day but don't let him fill himself up and reduce his appetite. At the same time, if he drinks rarely but otherwise seems healthy then don't worry, you can be sure that he's simply a baby who doesn't get very thirsty. You can use a bottle or a cup but don't allow him to get used to having all his drinks in bottles, as he'll tend to use it as a comforter and be constantly drinking to the detriment of his teeth. There's nothing else

suitable for a baby under 12 months – soft drinks, tea and coffee are out.
See also DEHYDRATION

DUCTS

See BLOCKED DUCTS

DUMMIES, SOOTHERS OR PACIFIERS

This is a topic more suited to books on general baby care and so if you want a discussion on whether dummies are revoltingly unattractive germ carriers or heaven's answer to a mother's prayer, then don't read on! I'd just like to add that it's funny how such innocent looking pieces of plastic can engender such strong feelings of passion and hatred ... However, there are issues related to feeding in the dummy debate. Firstly, it's not widely known among mothers that the safety of the rubber used in dummies and TEATS has come under international scrutiny in recent years. It's primarily because the chemicals (nitrosamines) used to preserve the rubber from rotting have been shown to cause stomach cancer in animals. This has led countries such as Germany and the United States to revise the maximum permitted levels of nitrosamines in dummies and teats, and manufacturers in other countries – like the UK and other EEC countries – have been looking at their products in the light of this. It has to be said that in organising experiments on animals, it is difficult to reproduce the effect of sucking on a dummy. The rubber is mixed with saliva, it may be sucked on for a few minutes a day or else many hours, for a few weeks or several years. The point is that we don't know, and won't ever be able to guarantee that dummies (and teats) are not a health hazard to babies. The risk that we run is never going to be huge or surely we'd have noticed something more concrete by now, and again it's up to you as a parent to work out how far it influences you.

The other aspect of dummy-use that relates to feeding lies in the fact that babies find sucking very comforting. A breastfed baby may get as much 'comfort sucking' as he needs at the breast, especially if he's allowed to feed as often as he wants to. A bottlefed baby may suck less than a breastfed baby, and may

75

therefore miss out on 'comfort sucking' and a dummy might fill the gap and keep him happier. Breastfed babies are sometimes very 'sucky' too, and a dummy is a useful way of soothing your baby if you're sure he needs it, and it's not possible for you to have him at your breast as often as he'd like. Nevertheless, this approach is not without risk to your MILK SUPPLY if you have a baby who isn't gaining and growing as he should. The dummy gives the baby sucking pleasure, and it's been known that some babies (especially small ones, who have less energy to yell for feeds) suck on a dummy instead of asking for a feed, and the mother thinks her baby is sleeping contentedly, on a full tummy. The truth is the baby is actually underfed and so the dummy needs to go in order for the baby to start demanding feeds more often. Similarly, if you're concerned about increasing your milk supply, and your baby uses a dummy, you'll need to discard it, so your baby gets all his sucking comfort from you. Your milk supply will increase as a result.

See STERILISING

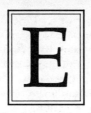

E

ECZEMA

Eczema is a skin condition, varying in severity from a few scaly or flaky patches of skin in one or two small areas of the body, to unsightly, itchy, sometimes weeping flaky skin all over the body. It's more common in bottlefed babies, which is one good argument for breastfeeding, and it's often associated with FOOD INTOLERANCE or ALLERGY to non-food items like soap or detergent. Fully breastfed babies can get eczema too, and latest research suggests that babies like this may be reacting to items of food coming through in the mother's milk. It could be that identifying the 'trigger' in the mother's diet helps to keep the condition at bay (see DIET AND BREASTFEEDING). It is extremely difficult to do this, and to be sure of being correct. Eczema quite naturally comes and goes, without obvious causes. When it comes to mixed feeding, certain foods seem to trigger-off eczema in susceptible babies, so if your baby has been diagnosed as having the condition it's definitely worthwhile making a note of what he eats and then comparing this with the condition of the eczema (see also DIET). If you get something that looks like a trigger, then excluding or reducing may be better for your baby than constant applications of steriod creams that do nothing about the underlying causes. Common culprits include eggs, milk, wheat and dairy products. Bear in mind, however, that dietary causes are difficult to pinpoint. Some doctors have expressed genuine concern that babies may go underfed, so if you want to explore the possibility of food exacerbating your baby's eczema, then do so with specialist help.

EGGS*

Another one of nature's own convenience foods, eggs are available everywhere, and they are quick and easy to prepare as well as being nourishing. Whole eggs – the white and the yoke – are a source of protein, fat, minerals (including iron) and vitamins. Their disadvantage is that they are often associated with ALLERGY, so they do need to be introduced gradually. Egg is an unsuitable food for babies at the start of mixed feeding; the white in particular needs to be introduced later than the yolk, because it is more likely to cause problems. Start your baby off on egg by giving tiny amounts of cooked yolk – boiled soft or hard, coddled or poached, it doesn't matter – mixed in with something else you know he's used to. Then build up on this, until you're sure he has no reaction to yolk. Seven months or so would be fine for most babies to start on whole eggs, the white included. If you suspect or know your child is food intolerant hold off the egg yolk until your baby is a year, and the white until he can tolerate the yolk without symptoms (see also FOOD INTOLERANCE). Small pieces of hard boiled egg make good finger food, or you can cut up an omlette into squares.

When? From the second stage of WEANING for the yolk; from seven months for whole egg.

ENGORGEMENT

This is a common breastfeeding problem, and it can happen at any time, though it's especially associated with the very early days. Engorged breasts are hard, swollen, enlarged and uncomfortable. A typical time is on the third or fourth day after delivery, when the COLOSTRUM changes to breast milk which is produced in larger quantities. As well as producing more milk, the breasts experience a greatly increased blood and lymph supply, and it's these factors that cause the swelling. If you've fed your baby frequently in the days before your milk 'comes in', as this change-over is called, you may only notice a slight change if anything at all. Your baby has simply taken the extra milk as and when you've produced it. I have heard mothers say that although their babies sucked and sucked in the first days, their milk 'never came in' and they had to stop breastfeeding as a result. This is a sad result of poor information, as probably their milk came in so beautifully and smoothly that they were never even aware of it.

Many babies, for whatever reason (sleepiness, jaundice, illness, a stay in a special care unit, for example) just don't feed very much at all in the first days and if they don't perk up by the time your milk is in, then you could get engorged. The basic treatment is to feed the baby. If your breasts need softening before he is LATCHING ON properly, then try EXPRESSING BREAST MILK by hand in order for this to happen. Massage, a warm bath, hot and cold compresses will start the flow if it's difficult to get going. Thereafter, feed as soon as your breasts become uncomfortable again. If your baby still isn't co-operating, then you will have to express more fully, emptying the breast by using the most efficient way for you. This may be by hand or with an electric pump (see BREAST PUMPS). There is a worry among some people that expressing from engorged breasts only makes the problem worse because it encourages the breasts to produce more milk. However, it's important to reduce the pressure from within the breast, as severe engorgement can lead to too much pressure, and then damage the milk producing cells. Allowing the milk, and the pressure, to subside allows normality to be restored within the breast and brings tremendous relief to the mother. Wear a well-supporting bra if you experience engorgement as this will keep you more comfortable (see BRAS).

In most cases, the baby starts to get hungrier and more active, and keeps pace with his mother's milk supply. The problem then solves itself. If this doesn't happen, and you go on becoming engorged, then you may be producing TOO MUCH MILK, and need to take the appropriate action. Don't allow your baby to go too long between feeds, or your breasts will become tense and swollen again, and possibly engorged. This is liable to happen at any time, if your baby sleeps longer than he usually does or if you are trying to wean him off the breast. Gentle hand-expressing will relieve the discomfort, as will feeding him, of course (see WEANING).

Women who don't want to breastfeed will experience engorgement in the early days. Keeping the breasts well-supported, perhaps with a binder round them and over the shoulders, and avoiding all but the gentlest expressing to relieve tension, so that the production of milk stops in a few days.

EQUIPMENT

Blenders, grinders and food processors are not essential but they are extremely useful when preparing food for all the family. You can chop or purée your baby's food to the variety of textures that she can cope with, very quickly. It is possible to buy a manual blender specially made for a baby: the serving dish is part of the blender and the food appears as you operate it. The usefulness of this is limited to the first few months, until your baby can wield a spoon and feed herself. A food processor is much better value, but as with all these things, you waste quite a bit of food, so you need to make largish quantities – great if you've got a freezer or twins with huge appetites! They're tricky to clean too, but certainly more efficient than a fork or sieve.

Pressure cookers can be used when preparing food for your baby, though as they are usually so big, one baby-sized portion of food isn't going to cover the bottom of the pan. Again, use it to make bigger quantities for freezing or for meals which the whole family can share in. Most people find the pressure cooker is very useful for cooking pulses which otherwise take a very long time. Pressure cooking allows the vitamin content of foods to be retained better than boiling, although if you always boil food in as little water as possible, and retain any cooking water left for gravy or soup, this isn't such an important point.

EXPRESSING BREAST MILK

You might need to do this for a number of reasons; your baby may be separated from you because of illness; he may have a defect (such as CLEFT LIP/PALATE) which makes normal breast-feeding difficult; or you may be suffering from engorgement; or else you may want to express because you're going out or working when you'd otherwise expect to feed. If you need to express a lot, perhaps to fulfil your baby's feeding needs for a long time, say at least a week, then it's certainly worth buying or hiring a breast pump. If you are expressing and not feeding directly at all, then you will need to express *at least* six times a day

80

in order to establish and maintain a milk supply. Expressing works like breastfeeding (though not normally as efficiently): the more you express, the more milk you'll produce. If you're partially expressing and partially feeding, then the total number of times your breasts need to be expressed and fed from, will need to be *at least* six, too (see BREAST PUMPS). If you are just collecting milk in order to have enough for an occasional feed then obviously these strictures won't apply. You can express whenever it's convenient for you. Some women find they have more milk in the morning, and can express after their baby's first feed of the day. Others find they always have plenty of milk in their breasts after a feed and use that time. Others do it between feeds.

Always express into a clean, sterilised container (see STERI-LISING). You can then transfer to another clean, sterilised container which you keep in the fridge. You can add to this store for 24 hours which is the longest recommended time for storing breast milk – unless you freeze it, in which case you can keep it there for three months. How much to express? That's a difficult one, as no one can predict how much milk a breastfed baby can take at any one feed. I can give you a very general rule of thumb, though: babies between seven and ten pounds will need around four ounces of EBM (expressed breast milk) per feed; babies between ten pounds and 12 pounds will need five ounces; babies between 12 pounds and 15 pounds will need seven ounces. Thereafter, reckon on eight ounces a feed. If you express regularly, you'll get to know your baby's needs more reliably.

Hand expressing is a lot less fiddly than expressing with a pump because there's nothing to sterilise (though obviously you'll make sure your hands are clean). There's also evidence that once you've got the hang of it, it's more effective at keeping up the milk supply than pumping. However, some women never manage to get more than a few drops however they express – it's no reflection on your milk supply, just on your expressing technique! If you don't get much with a pump, try with your hands and vice versa.

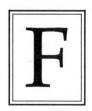

FAMILY MEALS

Once your baby is on solid foods, you may still feel it's easier to give her meals separately from the adults and other children, if there are any, in the household. After all, you can enjoy your own meal more peacefully if your baby's had her fill or if she's sleeping in another room. But it's a good experience to have a proper family meal when you can fit it in. Babies are so sociable, and really enjoy meals with other people, that it's worth compromising your routine, and your child's, in order to sit round the table together. Give her finger food that she can pop in her mouth herself, bring her chair up to the table, or else take the tray off and push the chair in so she can eat at the table too, and she'll enjoy being a part of the mealtime gathering. If this is difficult for you to do at every meal, or even every day, try to make it a feature of the weekends. Don't worry about table manners at this stage – your baby's too young to understand them and too young to remember them. Just give her food that's as un-messy as you can make it if you're concerned about her flinging it around. Obviously, you'll show you don't like her throwing stuff on the floor or over her head, but she's bound to do it for a little while yet.

FAMILY DOCTOR/GP

See HELP AND ADVICE

FAT

Fats in foods provide a concentrated source of energy, and in an infant, polyunsaturated fatty acids ensure the correct development of the brain and nervous system. In adults, it's thought that too high a proportion of saturated fat (mainly from animal sources) in the diet can lead to heart and circulatory problems. The advice is to replace these fats with unsaturated fats (mainly from vegetable sources). WEANING your baby onto a healthy diet means paying attention to fat and avoiding a diet that has too much. Fatty foods, including fried food, should be kept to a minimum, not just because of concern about a healthy diet for the future, but also because a baby's digestive system is not yet mature enough to cope with large amounts. Don't feel that today's emphasis on low-fat diets means you should give your baby skimmed or semi-skimmed milk, however (see COW'S MILK). The fat here is needed for energy, and for the vitamins it contains. Some children have METABOLIC DISORDERS that prevent them digesting fats. This will show up as failure to thrive, and fatty greasy stools.

FATHERS & BREASTFEEDING

Occasionally, fathers are unhappy about the idea of their partners BREASTFEEDING. It may be to do with the embarrassment at the possibility of others seeing; it may be to do with sexual jealousy; it may be that he wants to have a close relationship with the baby and resents the closeness that breastfeeding represents. This is why you do need to ask your partner how he feels about feeding – and try to get him to be honest. Breastfeeding's not always easy and natural from the word 'go', and support from your partner is essential. In that sense, he's important to the breastfeeding experience, just as you are. Let him know that no one needs to see much at all when you're breastfeeding. You may need to reassure him that breastfeeding won't mean you can't share your breasts with him as part of your sexual life together (see SEX AND BREASTFEEDING). However, it's true that some women do feel awkward about their breasts having a sexual role as well as a 'feeding role'. Think about whether you feel this way, too. Resolving not to let these feelings take you over is part of being an adult. As for the idea that somehow you will steal a march on the baby-parent relationship by breastfeeding, explain that feeding is only one part of baby care. He can become involved in other ways – cuddling, rocking, dressing and changing, bathing, pram-pushing, walking with baby in a sling . . . the list goes on! In any case, the time when your baby is exclusively breastfed, relying on that alone for food, comfort and security, is very short, when you consider the length of his childhood as a whole. No one's ever found that breastfed children relate any better or worse to their fathers as a result of that early feeding experience. People often joke that breastfeeding's better for dads, as there's no possibility of them having to get up to do the night feeds! And many men positively enjoy seeing their partners breastfeed. Your man may start off being negative – and come round to the idea once he sees it in practice. Then when your baby's on mixed feeding, fathers can be involved as much as they want, of course.

FEEDING–STAGES IN THE FIRST YEAR

In the first week   Some babies feed infrequently in the first day or two after birth – others are very keen, right from the start. Make sure you have your baby well-positioned on the nipple (see also LATCHING ON), and simply offer him feeds when he seems restless or distressed. Offer both sides at each feed, but allow him to suck on the first one as long as he wants to before offering him the other, and don't worry if he doesn't seem to want much on that second one. The next time, begin the feed on the opposite side to the one you started on previously.

During this first week, your baby will change day by day. He may start to feed much more frequently from the third day or so on, for example. He's quite likely to want to be breastfeeding eight or 10 times a day – but you'll get on better if you don't even think about counting or timing! The exception to this would be with a sleepy, small or underweight or ill baby; you may need to wake a baby like this in order to make sure he feeds frequently enough to be nourished, and frequently enough to stimulate your MILK SUPPLY. Not all mothers, not even all second-, third- and fourth-timers, reach the stage of easy, confident breastfeeding by the end of this week. Some babies are still slow to latch on properly, for example. Some mothers are still suffering from ENGORGEMENT or soreness. The point is that it's still early days as far as breastfeeding's concerned. It's great if everything is going well by this time, but it's far from being a disaster if it isn't. Just be patient, seek help if you need it, and remind yourself, when things aren't going as well as you had thought they might, that they will work out in the end. Don't feel you need to 'build up' from short breastfeeds to longer ones during this week. Elsewhere in this book I describe why limiting feeds according to set number of 'minutes per side' is likely to work against the establishment of happy breastfeeding (see DEMAND FEEDING). Nevertheless, mothers are often advised to start off with a minute a side on the first day, increasing to two minutes on the second day or whatever. There is no rational basis for this advice. Comparative studies have shown that it *doesn't* prevent sore nipples, which are likely to be caused by poor positioning, and in any case it's totally unworkable. How do you know when two minutes are up? It can take all of that and more to get sucking comfortably in these early days and then he's likely to stop and start. Do you count up the number of seconds he appears to have sucked and add them up . . .?

Bottle feeding babies may adopt a similar sort of pattern to breastfed babies – a couple of days of feeding infrequently, followed by an increase in demand. However, a bottle fed baby is more likely to go longer between feeds because some formula milk takes longer to digest, and because he's probably offered a similar amount at each feed, and encouraged to finish it. It may also be because mothers who choose to bottle feed may be more concerned about scheduled feeds. This pattern may not yet have established itself by the end of the first week, however. With both breast and bottle fed babies, it's usual for day and night to be undifferentiated and so your baby is no more likely to sleep longer at night than at any other time.

See also FIRST FEED

In the first month By the end of the first month, breastfeeding is usually going smoothly. Some babies are already spacing their feeds out, and adopting more predictable ROUTINES. Night feeds are the norm, though you'll probably find that if your baby does have a time when he's likely to go without a feed for more than three hours or so, it's at night. Wakefulness in the evening is very common during this month and some babies like to be near or on the breast very frequently, even those who have started to go longer between feeds at other times of the day or night. Don't be tempted to give top-ups of formula milk in the evenings. This will undermine your milk supply and may lead to other problems (see COMPLEMENTARY & SUPPLEMENTARY BOTTLES; FOOD INTOLERANCE).

Bottlefed babies are probably on six feeds a day by the end of the first month. You may have also started to give your baby the occasional drink of water between bottle feeds. Your baby is likely to need at least one feed during the night, and possibly two.

One month to six months Breastfed babies can continue to feed on the breast exclusively throughout this time, as long as their growth is satisfactory. By the end of this time, the baby becomes a truly expert feeder, often finishing the feed after only one side or after just a few minutes on one or both breasts. He may continue to have the occasional long feed, however, especially in the evening. Some babies drop all night feeds at sometime between two months and six months, though it's not uncommon for a baby to still need them. Try waking your baby at 11 or so when you go to bed yourself, if she doesn't wake by herself. This may allow her to go through the night without disturbing you. Then later, you can try dropping that very late feed altogether.

Frequent feeding is probably a thing of the past by the end of this time, though all babies have the odd few days here and there when they seem to need to feed frequently again. This is perfectly normal. It may be that they're extra hungry; it may be that they need to 'tell' your milk supply to increase; it may be that they need the milk to help fight against an infection. If your baby seems to need extra milk, and more frequent feeding doesn't seem to satisfy her, then you can think about trying a few tiny tastes of solid food before six months (see WEANING).

Bottlefed babies may need solids from about four to four and a half months, though not all do. Some are perfectly happy on formula milk alone for longer. Most bottle fed babies are down to five bottles a day by the time they reach four to four and a half months, and it may be better to increase their range of foods rather than increase the formula intake. Night feeds are still common, though if you are giving a full bottle of milk when your baby wakes up in the night, think about offering WATER instead, or else just a small amount of milk, if feeding is the only way to settle your baby.

Six months to a year   By the end of the first year, most babies, breast and bottle fed, will be joining in family meals, or at least having breakfast, lunch and tea based on the diet the rest of the family follows. Drinks will come in a cup for most babies, though plenty of babies still enjoy breastfeeding too. Most babies who've been bottle fed still have at least an evening bottle to help them get to sleep. Remember that formula milk and breast milk rather than ordinary full-fat pasturised milk, are better for babies until at least a year (see MILK). Your baby will have developed certain likes and dislikes, and she'll even be happy to start playing around with a spoon, attempting to feed herself, although most babies don't actually manage anything efficient until much later. Food fads and battles over mealtimes are a feature of the toddler years and their foundations can start before 12 months. Don't get cross with your baby if she doesn't want to eat her dinner. Don't get involved in 'pacts' like trying to get her to eat her vegetables before you'll let her have the yoghurt you know she loves. Keep mealtimes happy and relaxed; serve your baby the food she likes, increasing her range with tastes of food which are new to her from time to time. Don't get too worried if she seems slow to take to solids, even at a year. Just keep working at it without becoming anxious, and get your health visitor's or doctor's reassurance that she's growing well and remaining healthy. See WEANING.

FIBRE

The outer cell walls of plants provide our diet with fibre, or 'roughage' as it was called when I was a child. It's now known that highly refined, relatively fibre-free diets can mean constipation at the very least, and severe bowel disease at the worst. It is better for most of us to include fresh fruit and vegetables in our diet, together with wholegrains (see CEREALS), as these are more likely to provide us with the fibre we need to stay healthy than processed, overcooked foods and 'white' grains. For babies on mixed feeding, the situation isn't quite like that. Foods with a lot of fibre – say, uncooked vegetables, or high-fibre breakfast cereals – are quite hard for a baby to digest. He can't chew very efficiently, so his saliva doesn't get a chance to start work on breaking down the food, and remember, his digestive system is used to milk only. If the food you're offering your baby is high in fibre, then it may need to be chopped or mashed into small pieces, or mixed with some liquid until he gets a little older and more able to cope. Fruit such as apples and pears should be peeled. However, it's a good start if your baby gets used to enjoying vegetables that haven't been cooked to a pulp and eats breakfast cereals that are free from sugar and made with the whole of the grain. Also that he has wholemeal bread and learns the different textures of food that's closer to its natural, more fibrous state.

FINGER FOOD*

Anything your baby manages to eat himself, without you popping it into his mouth for him, is a finger food. Babies enjoy the experience of this little bit of independence; it's an excellent way for them to learn about the different textures and appearances of foods; and above all it's a really convenient 'feeding method' for you. For me, one of the most powerful arguments in favour of delaying solids until six months or so, is that a baby is then able to feed himself to a large extent, if you give him the right sorts of food. This is quite a plus point, especially if you have a toddler or other older children who inevitably need some of your attention at mealtimes as well. It gives you a chance to get on with some of your own meal while it's still hot, too.

You'll get plenty of ideas for finger food throughout this book, but a collection of popular suggestions would include: banana slices or cubes; apple slices; pear slices; rusks; toast; bread; vegetables sliced or in fingers, such as carrot, potato; peas; small pieces of meat; non-oily fish, cut up into pieces. You do need to make sure that the food you're giving your baby is in small pieces but they do need to be big enough for him to pick up. Soft-textured food is best unless the food can be sucked to a manageable pulp, like toast or rusks. Food that's hard, like raw carrot is too difficult for babies to cope with without good chewing and gnawing skills. Of course, you'll always make sure you stay with your baby when he's eating finger food, because of the risk of CHOKING.

FIRST FEED

These days, it's more and more usual to offer your baby his first breastfeed as soon after delivery as you want to – more or less straight away, if you and he are in 'good condition' after the birth and most mothers and babies are. There's a sound physiological basis for doing this as the hormone OXYTOCIN is released in response to the baby's sucking. This encourages the blood vessels in the uterus to contract and expel the placenta, which completes the third stage of labour. Most women delivering in western hospitals get a routine injection of the synthetic hormone syntometrine, just as the baby is born. This acts almost immediately on the uterus, and the placenta is expelled relatively quickly in these circumstances; the oxytocic effect of the first feed is very largely irrelevant. More and more women and midwives are questioning the benefits of an actively-managed third stage, however. They prefer to allow the placenta to come away naturally, under the influence of natural oxytocin, helped in part by the stimulation of the first feed.

Whether or not you want to have an actively-managed third stage, you can still enjoy the positive effects of feeding your baby as soon as he's born. Cuddle your baby close to your breast, and allow him to take the nipple if he shows an interest in it. Some babies are interested in feeding straight away. Others may take half an hour or more to seem keen. Don't hurry your baby or feel under pressure yourself. It may be that your baby will just prefer to smell and lick your nipple, rather than actually feed. It doesn't matter. These moments of greeting are just as precious. Mothers who give their babies a first feed while still in the delivery room are likely to breastfeed for longer but this may reflect their motivation and keenness to breastfeed as well as the physical effect of getting breastfeeding underway good and soon. Don't worry if your baby has to be taken into special care after birth, or if you're too exhausted and zonked out with fatigue and/or pain relievers to even think about feeding. Time and patience later on, plus support and help in the early days and whenever necessary, are far more potent factors in successful breastfeeding. If the first feed doesn't happen soon, for whatever reason, simply offer your baby a feed just as soon as you can. And bottle feeding mothers should do the same, give a bottle in the delivery room if you wish to, or else soon after.

FISH*

Fish has been traditionally thought of as 'brain food', I suppose because of its high concentrations of some of the B vitamins. It doesn't play as great a part in people's diets as it used to for no obvious reason, but recent trends indicate an upsurge in fish-eating so perhaps there's a genuine revival in store. Fish is a useful source of protein, vitamins and minerals, and many varieties are just right for babies. Much fish is quick and easy to prepare, too. You can start your baby on fish once he's got used to mixed feeding, and is able to enjoy small amounts of foods such as rice, fruit and vegetables without problems, unless you have a good reason to suspect FOOD INTOLERANCE, in which case you should wait until your baby's a year or so. First tastes of fish should be small, and be of a white, non-oily variety such as cod or coley. This is because oily fish (like herring) may be too fatty for your baby's digestion at first (see also FAT). Obviously, you need to make sure all the fishbones are taken out before you serve it to your baby. It's understandable to be worried about bones in fish – after all, it can be difficult to be absolutely positive you've got every last little bone out. One way round this is to choose a fish with very obvious bones in it, such as monk fish or trout. Or serve fish in fish cakes that you've mixed in a food processor. That way, tiny bones will be ground up and they'll be too small to cause a problem.

Once your baby's happy on white fish, you can try her on other types, including tinned fish, but avoid the sorts that are actually tinned in oil, like some brands of sardines or pilchards. Tinned tuna and tinned salmon are usually liked by babies. Shellfish should be avoided because it may contain high levels of pollutants and/or toxic trace elements. What about fish fingers? If you avoid brands with colouring in the coating (read the label), and grill them instead of frying, then fish fingers are fine. They avoid the problem of fishbones, and if you chop them up they can be eaten very easily as finger food (see ADDITIVES AND COLOURINGS).

When? From the second stage of WEANING.

90

FLAT NIPPLES

See NIPPLES

FLOUR*

Most flour used in this country is wheat flour. Wheat flour contains GLUTEN, and this is often associated with ALLERGY. For this reason, it's not a good idea to introduce wheat flour in any form, for example in bread and other baked goods or as a thickener for soups or other dishes, until your baby is happy on gluten-free cereals (such as rice), fruit and vegetables. You can buy flour made from other cereals if you need to use flour in cooking for your baby before he reaches this stage – rice flour is probably the most widely available. Once you've decided to introduce wheat flour into your baby's diet, remember that wholemeal flour uses the whole of the grain and it's therefore more nutritious. Other wholegrain flours are good for baking, too – granary flour and rye flour give different tastes and textures.

FLUID INTAKE

See DRINKS

FOOD INTOLERANCE

Throughout this book, I've tended to use the term 'food intolerance' to describe any adverse reaction to a food item or group of food items. It's a more useful term, especially to the layperson, than food allergy. ALLERGY, strictly speaking, involves the immune system, however there are disorders whose symptoms are brought on by certain foods that don't involve the immune system at all.

When it has an allergic reaction to a food, the body produces symptoms that are a direct result of contact with the 'offending' substance, or 'allergen'. The body has previously been sensitised to the substance. This can happen as a result of a deficiency in the immune system (and this deficiency may be something the subject is born with), or else he may have been bottle fed and therefore not received the substance immunoglobulin A ('IgA') in the BREAST MILK, or else he may have had an illness that has damaged the lining of the intestine (that would otherwise protect him against this sensitising response). The next time the child meets the allergen, the antibodies that formed at the first encounter, swing into action again and cause what we term an allergic response. In other forms of food intolerance, the sorts that do not involve the immune system, the body is unable to cope with certain foods, or certain constituents in them. The disorders are caused by a 'fault' in the digestive system itself, such as an inability to produce a digestive enzyme. Intolerance covers both sorts of response, so it's a useful catch-all term.

Over recent years, doctors and dieticians have come to accept that food intolerance is more common than we once thought and that it can be responsible for a wider range of symptoms in babies, children and adults. It's a fertile area for research, and as more answers are found, more questions are raised. The very existence of food intolerance has implications for the way mothers are advised to feed their babies. No one knows exactly how high a proportion of babies and children may be food intolerant, though I have seen estimates of ten per cent. What is clear is that symptoms such as COLIC, CRYING and restlessness in babies sometimes clear up when attention is paid either to the baby's diet or the mother's (see DIET; DIET AND BREASTFEED-ING). ECZEMA and asthma are more common in babies who are bottle fed, or, more specifically, in babies who have not been exclusively breastfed for the first four to six months of life. Babies who suffer from colic may go on to develop other symptoms of food intolerance. COELIAC DISEASE is more common in babies who were artificially fed, and/or who had early solids. The body of respectable scientific literature that demonstrates the link between diet and a range of disorders in childhood such as epilepsy and migraine, is growing.

Many specialists in the field of infant nutrition are convinced that breastfeeding is vitally important in preventing the develop-ment of food intolerance, or in helping to reduce its severity. The rise in artificial feeding in the last thirty years or so has gone hand-in-hand with increased food intolerance, and in fact, FORMULA MILK (or anything but breast milk) is so very different in its effect on our physiology – the digestive system and the immune system – that we cannot know its full extent, despite the fact that most artificially fed infants appear to thrive well enough.

It's not the purpose of this book to discuss the full extent of food intolerance. However, we do know that babies of parents with food intolerance themselves, or babies who have one or more close relatives with eczema, asthma or severe hay fever, are more susceptible to the tendency. Therefore it makes sense for you to breastfeed your baby without supplements for at least the first four to six months, when your baby's immune and digestive systems are more likely to be mature enough to cope. When solids are introduced, introduce them gradually, avoiding the most common sources of intolerance until later on (see also WEANING). You'll see the appropriate information about 'when' under the headings for different foods. Bear in mind that there may be many reasons other than food intolerance for disorders which affect your baby, these may be, as above, eczema, asthma or hay fever.

Whether you're breast or bottle feeding, and your baby seems to be unhappy or else doesn't thrive, consider the possibility of food intolerance, and ask your doctor for referral to a specialist. Failure to thrive linked with refusal of feeds and/or severe vomiting, is far more common in bottle fed babies, though it can occur, very occasionally, in breastfed babies, too. It can be helped by looking at the sort of milk the baby is having, if bottle fed. Sometimes a change to SOYA MILK helps (though babies who are food intolerant to COW'S MILK may also be intolerant to soya milk). The soya milk used must be a type specially modified for babies. You may also want to think about relactation (see also CHANGING FROM BOTTLE TO BREAST). If you're breastfeeding, think about your own diet. These measures should be taken as well as getting your baby investigated for some underlying disorder or illness. Babies on solids can display signs of food intolerance, too. A baby who seems slow at taking to solids needs to be allowed to go at his own pace. Watch for signs of a reaction to any new food. Common foods that cause reactions include wheat, eggs, milk (non-human), citrus fruits, fish, food with additives and colourings. We all need to know a lot more about food intolerance.

See BOOKLIST

FOOD PROCESSOR

See EQUIPMENT

FOOD REFUSAL

It sometimes happens that a baby refuses solid foods. If this is the case with your baby, think about the following possibilities:
• you're offering SOLIDS at too young an age. Four to six months is the standard time but by no means all babies need solids at this age. His rejection of the solid food may be his only way of letting you know that he isn't ready yet. Give it a rest for a week or two before trying again.
• he's not hungry for them at this particular time. Try another time of the day for his first tastes.
• he's too keen on the breast or bottle to want the new experience of solids. Try 'sandwiching' his solids between 'sides' of a breastfeed, or two halves of his bottle (see WEANING).
• he doesn't like the taste of what you're offering him. Try mixing first tastes with expressed breast milk (see EXPRESSING BREASTMILK) or formula milk to make the new taste less unfamiliar.
• he can't manage large quantities. Give him no more than the tiniest smidgin at a time, on the end of the spoon.
• he's already having to get used to other new experiences, perhaps a move to a cot from a crib, being looked after by a childminder or moving house, and solids are another he could do without! Again, leave it for a couple of weeks before trying again.
• what you are offering doesn't agree with him. Go back to foods you know he has taken before, or else check that what you're starting him on is suitable. Go slowly on introducing new foods.
• your baby is ill or a little off colour (see ILLNESS).
• your baby is TEETHING and needs the comfort of the breast or bottle.
• your baby's uncomfortable in the way he's sitting. Try him on your knee or else in a different sort of chair (for example, a bouncing cradle rather than a high chair) until he gets used to solids.

- she's drinking several bottles of milk a day, which takes away her appetite for solid food.
- she hates being spoonfed. Give her finger foods instead.
- she doesn't like the texture of the foods you're giving her.

Don't get anxious if your baby's slow to take to solids or shows a dislike of certain foods. Making mealtimes happy and anxiety-free is an important point which will help avoid battles at the table during the coming toddler years.

See also BREAST REFUSAL

FORE MILK

BREAST MILK is not consistently uniform. One of the major differences lies between HIND MILK which is further inside the breast and which is made available to the baby by the LET-DOWN REFLEX and fore milk, which is stored in the reservoirs behind the nipple and areola. It's the fore milk that the baby sucks when he first gets to the breast, which 'keeps him going' until the let-down reflex allows the hind milk to be released into the ducts leading to the nipple. It is lower in fat, and therefore calories, than hind milk and so babies who only get fore milk tend not to put on weight so well. The reason for a baby only getting fore milk may be because the mother's let-down reflex doesn't work efficiently or because the mother switches the baby to the other side too quickly, before the baby has had time to milk the first breast sufficiently (there's normally no need to decide for your baby when to change sides – let him reach a natural break before you change over).

FORMULA MILK

Sometimes known as 'baby milk', formula milk is the accepted international term for non-human milk that has been prepared for consumption by human infants. It refers, almost always, to cow's milk, that has been modified by an industrial process. Among other changes, it alters the fat, sodium and protein levels of cow's milk to make it more suitable for a human infant. Breast milk can't be reproduced, however, and there are constituents of it, such as ANTIBODIES, that protect a baby against infection, illness and ALLERGY that would seem unlikely ever to be developed artificially. It's rather like trying to develop artificial blood or gastric juices or lymph. These are all living fluids, not laboratory-made ones.

The history of artificial feeding is a fascinating one – babies have been given all sorts of different foods other than breast milk. It's not a very comforting one, however (see BOOKLIST). Babies throughout history have died or been harmed because of being fed other than on the breast. Certain foods, and milks, which we now know are totally unsuitable for human infants have been promoted as equal to, and in some cases superior to, mothers' milk. Even in the last few years, quite important changes have been made to formula milk as a result of new discoveries about breast milk. The fact is that finding a substitute for breast milk is not an easy task, and the more we know about breast milk, the more difficult it is. To give one example out of many, the substance Taurine was discovered in breast milk in the early 1980s. It was shown to be important for the full development of the nervous system and the brain. So, formula manufacturers put it in their infant formulas. What about the infants fed on taurine-deficient formula before then? Did it matter? Does it matter? What if the taurine now present in infant formula depends on some other substance *not* in formula but present in breast milk, in order for it to be fully absorbed by the infant's body? Will we know? We do know that the majority of bottle fed babies in the West appear to thrive and develop well on formula milk, and that work to develop and improve formula must continue, as there will always be a need for a breast milk substitute. It's only a minority who develop severe FOOD INTOLERANCE as a result of being formula fed (and because breast milk doesn't guarantee protection against intolerance, some of these babies may have been affected anyway). Other risks with formula milk are even less clear cut. All we can do is to observe that the digestive process is different in formula fed babies, that they miss out on certain aspects of breast milk, and note that on the whole, bottlefed babies, wherever they are, are more likely to fall ill than breastfed ones. This is a matter of life and death in the Third World, mainly because of the way mothers may not have access to clean water to make up the feeds, or because they dilute the powder too much to save money. In the West, the risk of poorly made up feeds is very small. But here, babies on formula milk are less well-protected against certain illnesses.

Formula milk is an industrial product. That's not to say it's automatically developed in a non-ethical way. But ingredients may be chosen that reflect economic priorities rather than health priorities. Moreover, despite health regulations, contamination can occur at any stage of the industrial process. Cows can be infected, milk can become infected in transit, and all the other ingredients that go into formula (such as coconut oil or artificially produced minerals and vitamins) may be less than perfect in some way. Occasionally, contaminated milk gets through (it happened in the UK with salmonella-infected Osterfeed at the beginning of the 1980s) but no one can say with certainty that mistakes are always discovered before they reach the consumer (that is, the baby). It's difficult to record these doubts without feeling worried about sounding unbalanced, or even scare-mongering. And I feel strongly that every mother should have a free choice as to how to feed her baby. Nevertheless, that choice can't be free unless it's informed. Until you know that there are areas of doubt about the suitability of formula in comparison with breast milk, you won't know the full implications of any choice you make.

Not all formula is based on cow's milk. Some is made from soya (see SOYA MILK), and is usually prescribed for babies who have a recognised cow's milk allergy. Other formulas are available for PRE-TERM BABIES. All these formulas have the same basic disadvantages outlined above, but they are useful for particular babies. You may find the formula your baby is on doesn't seem to suit her. She might appear unsettled and need feeding frequently or perhaps she's often sick. Ask your health visitor if your baby may be better off on a different sort. There are two basic types, one with modified cow's milk protein (which used to be known as 'humanised milk'), and the other with unmodified cow's milk protein. The second type generally takes longer to digest.

Follow-on milk (so-called) is a formula meant for older babies of at least four months of age. The iron content is higher than ordinary full-fat pasteurised milk, so it is considered to be better for a baby who may be about to make the change from ordinary baby formula.

FREEZER

Something over half the households in this country have the use of a freezer. Freezing food preserves it, with a very small loss of vitamins. It can be helpful to make use of your freezer when you have a baby to feed, and very organised households stock up the freezer with meals before the baby's born, so there's time afterwards to relax, rest, get to know the baby and get feeding established without the bother of cooking. If you manage to do this, congratulations and stop looking smug!

It's more likely you'll use the freezer after the birth. I think it's handy to always have a few loaves of bread in the freezer, so at least you never run out of that (of course you can forget to take it out in time for it to defrost before breakfast). More specifically where the baby's concerned, breast milk can be expressed and stored in the freezer for up to three months. If you're not very sure about how much to store for a feed it's helpful to store it in separate small quantities – a couple of ounces or so. Then, you don't run the risk of freezing a whole six or seven ounces, only for your baby-sitter or minder to defrost the whole lot and find the baby only takes an ounce or two. You'd then have to discard the unused milk; you can't refreeze it once it's been defrosted, warmed (by standing the bottle in a jug of water) and partially used. Doing this would run the risk of bugs growing in the milk. Some mothers actually freeze their milk in ice cube trays, decanting it into a bottle once it's defrosted (see EXPRESSING BREAST MILK). Meals for a baby on solid food can be made in large quantities and then frozen in meal-sized portions. Again, the ice-cube tray is useful here, especially when your baby's not eating much solid food. I have used ice cubes myself, stirred into the dinner. It's a quick way to cool food down that's too hot to give a baby who's nevertheless yelling with hunger and impatience, and unlike mixing it with water from the tap, it doesn't add too much liquid.

FRIDGE

If you are EXPRESSING BREAST MILK it will keep in the fridge for 24 hours, by which time you should either freeze it, use it or discard it. An unused portion of your baby's meal will be safe for the same amount of time (see LEFT-OVERS). Bottle feeding mothers find it useful to make up the whole day's feed in one go, either keeping it all in a large, lidded jug or else storing it in the appropriate number of bottles. Either way, the milk can then be warmed, if your baby prefers it warmed, by standing the bottle in a jug of hot water until it reaches the right temperature. Whatever you store in the fridge, make sure you keep it covered, so other bits and pieces don't fall in by mistake.

FROZEN FOOD

Bought frozen foods may be suitable for your baby, as long as you read the label information and avoid the ones with ingredients your baby isn't ready for, or ones which include ADDITIVES AND COLOURINGS. Frozen vegetables or frozen fruit should be fine for baby – there is a small quantity of vitamins lost in the freezing process, but that should be insignificant, as your baby's diet won't ever be composed entirely of frozen foods (see also CONVENIENCE FOODS; FREEZER).

FRUIT

Some fruits – notably pears, apples, bananas, among the sorts most widely available – are good first tastes for babies starting on mixed feeding. Fruits with seeds in such as strawberries should be left until the second stage of weaning, and citrus fruits should be delayed as well. Don't aim to introduce seeded or citrus fruit to a baby who you suspect of FOOD INTOLERANCE until 12 months as these fruits are associated with intolerance, and delaying their introduction may help your baby develop the ability to cope with them better. The fruit you offer your baby will need to be cooked or very finely grated at first (except for bananas, which mash easily), and always peeled. From the age of about six or seven months, or after you're sure he can cope with cooked fruit, your baby will enjoy small slices of raw fruit or larger grated pieces. Peeling is still advisable until the second year as the skin is usually too tough for a baby to chew through and digest efficiently.

Dried fruit makes a good finger food though it's sticky and sweet, so brush teeth afterwards. You can make JELLIES from fruit, or add pieces of it to yoghurt.

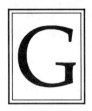

GASTROENTERITIS

The symptoms of gastroenteritis are VOMITING and DIAR-RHOEA, and the cause is an infection, bacterial or viral, within the digestive tract. Breastfed babies are virtually totally protected from the most common forms of gastroenteritis because of the ANTIBODIES present in breast milk. Bottle fed babies aren't protected, and bugs grow quickly in milk, which is why you need to observe the rules of STERILISING if you bottle feed. Contaminated food can cause food poisoning, and lead to diarrhoea and vomiting. You need to be careful about the food you use when your baby's on mixed feeding, too, and about the way you prepare it (see HYGIENE). Babies with tummy bugs can get worse more quickly than older children, and you need to ask your doctor's advice if the symptoms cause you concern.
See also DEHYDRATION

GELATINE

Gelatine is a product obtained from animal cartilage that's used to 'set' jellies, mousses and so on. The vegetarian product is based on seaweed and it's called agar agar. Either can be used in jellies or other dishes for your baby once you're sure your baby can cope with the fruit or whatever you're using on its own. Don't introduce a new food in gelatine.

GLUTEN

This is a protein found in certain cereals. It causes bread and pastry mixes to rise slightly and helps to bind ingredients together. Wheat contains gluten, as does rye, barley and oats but in lesser quantities. Gluten is often linked with FOOD INTOLER-

100

ANCE, and people with COELIAC DISEASE or with a sensitivity to gluten, need to follow a gluten-free diet, though they may be able to manage some of the cereals with less gluten than wheat. Babies starting on mixed feeding are better off avoiding gluten until they're able to tolerate gluten-free cereal such as rice. In practical terms, this means delaying the introduction of wheat-containing products, such as bread, wheat rusks and wheat or oat-based breakfast cereals. Some packaged baby foods have a gluten-free symbol on the label which is helpful.

GOAT'S MILK

In recent years there have been reports of babies and children with marked COW'S MILK intolerance being able to drink goat's milk, without problems. There's nothing especially 'better' about goat's milk. It's certainly not advisable to give it to babies under a year old unless you have medical approval for doing so. The reasons are that goat's milk is short of essential B vitamins. It may not be pasteurised, and unless you know the herd the milk comes from is well looked after and disease free, you do risk your baby catching an infection from contaminated milk. With older children this may not matter, as less of their diet is based on milk, and they are better able to cope with the occasional bug without becoming ill.

GOOSEBERRIES

See BERRIES

GRAINS

See CEREALS

GRAPES

Grapes are a suitable food for your baby from the second stage of WEANING. If you give them at this early stage, you'll need to wash them well and then either peel and chop them, discarding the pips, or else push them through a sieve. This is all rather fiddly, but until your baby is a lot older, he'll find the skins too

101

tough and both skins and pips hard to digest (he'll not be able to remove the pips himself for many a long month – or year!). Later on, grapes are good finger food (peeled and depipped). The small, sweet varieties are usually very popular, and because the skin is finer, you can leave small grapes unpeeled – though you will still have to cut them in half to enable your baby to chew them properly.

When? Peeled, depipped and chopped/sieved from the second stage of WEANING. As finger food, peeled and depipped, from nine months.

GRAPEFRUIT

Grapefruits are fine as a food for a baby, though they aren't suitable until the age of six months plus, like other citrus fruits. They are usually too tart for a baby's taste on their own. You can make a grapefruit purée, either on its own or with orange, and sweeten it with natural apple juice. Tiny pieces of grapefruit can be mixed with yoghurt, where its bitterness won't be noticed so much.

When? From the second stage of WEANING.

GREEN BEANS

Green beans, fresh or frozen (without ADDITIVES AND COLOURINGS) can be given to your baby once he's used to other, blander vegetables like potato and carrot. Chop them and give them as finger food after steaming or boiling (fast, in a small amount of water), or else mash or purée.

When? From the second stage of WEANING.

GROWTH OF BABY

See WEIGHT

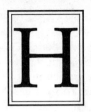

HAM

Ham is preserved pork, and because SALT is used in the preserving process, as well as other chemicals (for instance, nitrates) which are thought by some experts to be potentially harmful, it shouldn't be given to young babies. Older babies – nine months and over – should be able to cope with small quantities, unless you suspect possible FOOD INTOLERANCE, when you should delay ham until you're sure your baby is able to tolerate pork.

HANDICAPPED BABIES

Feeding a mentally or physically handicapped baby has special problems. It would be impossible to go through a list of particular difficulties here as so much depends on the specific handicap your baby may have. However, breastfeeding a handicapped baby may present a problem because the baby may have difficulties with muscular co-ordination that makes sucking on the nipple slow and unrewarding. Sleepiness, and general weakness leading to fatigue, may add to the problem. Sometimes, babies with a handicap that affects their ability to suck are helped with a special teat used on a bottle. You can then try EXPRESSING BREAST MILK and feeding that way. Write to the Disabled Living Foundation for information about feeding aids and equipment.
See BOOKLIST; USEFUL ADDRESSES

HEALTH VISITOR

See HELP AND ADVICE

103

HELP AND ADVICE

The sources of help and advice which you may seek for help with your baby's feeding problems are most likely to come from your family doctor, health visitor or midwife.

Family doctors may not know a great deal about baby feeding unless they have young children of their own or else they have made it an area of special personal interest. A paediatrician (a doctor specialising in the medical care of babies and children) may see your baby if she has feeding problems that lead to a failure to thrive or to develop normally. They are, or should be, expert in knowing whether a baby is growing well and this can be important, either to reassure you, or to confirm what is wrong if questions have been raised about your baby's weight.

Your health visitor or midwife is likely to have better information and advice concerning feeding, simply because she is trained to deal with this sort of thing in particular, and is used to the questions which mothers raise about feeding. In the UK, they are nurses with specialist qualifications. The midwife works either in hospital or outside as a 'community midwife'. Part of the midwife's training is concerned with helping new mothers to establish breastfeeding and overcome some of the common problems. Of course, you'll meet midwives during your pregnancy and you can ask any questions you have in advance. After the birth you'll normally see her for up to 28 days, so she won't be around to help you with weaning. Get the midwife to make sure your baby is well positioned at the breast if you are new to breastfeeding or if you have had problems before (see LATCH-ING ON; POSITION AT BREAST).

The health visitor takes over the care of you and your baby when the midwife 'signs you off', some days after the birth of your baby. This can be at any time between ten and 28 days. Normally your health visitor will visit you at home in the first few weeks, and there will also be routine health checks either at home or at a baby clinic. Visits to the clinic for weighing are also an opportunity to discuss non-medical questions such as feeding and general care. Not all health visitors are sufficiently well informed about breastfeeding to give practical and useful help. So, if your health visitor suggests bottle feeding and you are not happy with this advice, ask her if her suggested strategy is the only way. She may refer you to a colleague, or you can also speak to a breastfeeding counsellor. A good health visitor is likely to be a real friend to a new mother, sharing her information with you and boosting your confidence. She's the person to talk to if your baby suffers from wind or seems to be spotty; if you think your baby is getting too much or not enough solid food; whether you should change your brand of formula milk; if you need new recipe ideas. . . .

For help with breastfeeding on a mother to mother level, contact a National Childbirth Trust breastfeeding counsellor, a counsellor from the Association of Breastfeeding Mothers or a La Leche League leader. Breastfeeding counsellors are normally mothers who have been through a training to learn about the practical aspects of breastfeeding, and about the skills and approach needed to counsel other mothers with queries or problems. You can usually phone them at any time. On a more informal level you can get a lot of help from other parents. Toddlers groups (which usually welcome babies of all ages), a NCT postnatal group or any other 'gathering' of parents and babies are all good ways of getting support, swapping information and realising that other parents have problems and questions, too.

See USEFUL ADDRESSES

HERBS

Flavouring your baby's meals with herbs is fine as long as you use small amounts (see SEASONING). Cold herbal teas are a pleasant drink for babies taking foods other than breast or formula milk. They have no obvious advantage over water, though, unless you're using them medicinally. You'd need to consult a specialist book or a herbalist about this. The herbal teas and drinks marketed especially for babies may be high in sugar, so read the label, and they are no better for your baby than sweetened fruit juice. An infusion of tea made with fresh leaves is better and just as convenient. Don't give your baby a strong infusion, however, and stick to mild flavours like camomile.

HIGH CHAIRS

A baby can be fed or feed himself solid food on your lap, but this proves to be rather too messy an experience for most parents to contemplate as routine. From about six months, or whenever your baby starts having foods other than milk (see WEANING), he can be strapped into a high chair. He really is a lot safer if he has a proper harness over his shoulders, fastened behind his back, with the side straps of the harness clipped to anchorage straps on the chair itself. When buying new, look for a label indicating that the high chair conforms to British Standard number: 5799. Some chairs will not have a number, but this doesn't necessarily mean that they are unsafe, if they come from a store with a reputation to maintain. If you buy second hand, check for the major safety features: there should be rings to hold the anchorage straps; the chair should feel sturdy enough to withstand a lot of deliberate toddler wriggling; it should not have castors on the end of the legs (these allow a child to make his high chair mobile, and potentially dangerous, by pushing with his legs and arms against a wall or against other furniture). The most versatile high chairs have a removable tray, which can be lifted back or taken off to allow your baby to sit at the family table (check that the arm rests on the high chair don't prevent this; if the chair has them, they should be low enough to slide under your table). It's handy if the chair folds flat, ironing-board fashion, when not in use, although the very sturdiest tend not to do this, and you may prefer the look of more traditional styles that don't do it either. Bear in mind that although wooden high chairs look lovely, especially if they have interestingly carved outlines, compared to the more modern chrome and plastic models they are a headache to keep clean. Wooden seats aren't as comfortable, and you may need to put in a cushion either under the baby's bottom or behind his back.

Some high chairs have a table-and-chair option – you separate out the component parts when your baby has outgrown the straight high chair mode. When deciding what to buy, don't be too enthused by this feature, because for a start, you may need it as a high chair when/if your next baby arrives, and secondly, the tables tend to have a tiny surface area that toddlers find almost useless for most activities. Chairs that start life as a low chair for a small baby, and then fix onto a frame to become a feeding chair are useful. You can sometimes fix the chair to hang from the frame as a swing, although don't try to do this unless the chair and the frame have been designed with this option in mind.

An alternative to a high chair is a fold-up seat and back, with a frame that grips onto the upper and lower surface of most ordinary table tops. This is especially useful for travelling and visiting. You can also buy a sort of fabric feeding sling: the baby sits in it, and the long straps tie him firmly and safely onto a kitchen or dining chair. It folds away into your handbag when not in use, and you can wash it when it's dirty.

HIND MILK

The BREAST MILK that's stored in the lobes is known as the hind milk as opposed to the FORE MILK which is stored behind the nipple in little reservoirs. For the hind milk to become available to your baby, the tiny muscles keeping the milk in have to relax under the influence of the LET-DOWN REFLEX and this then releases the milk. It's important for your baby to get the hind milk, as it is rich in calories which will help your baby grow. Occasionally, babies who appear to be feeding frequently may not put on weight sufficiently because they are not getting enough hind milk. When this is the case, it sometimes turns out that the mother is deliberately taking the baby off the first breast, because she's anxious that there won't be time to 'fit in' the second breast before the baby loses interest in feeding. The result is that the baby doesn't manage to get his full quota of hind milk – and he's therefore liable to gain weight unacceptably slowly *and* be hungry again soon after each feed. The solution is to keep the baby at one breast until he appears satisfied, even if that means he zonks out on the breast without even nibbling at the second. Just remember to offer the 'unused' breast first at the next feed.

HOLIDAYS

Don't be put off having a holiday away from home just because you have a small baby. There are ways of making the whole feeding scene quite easy. If you're fully breastfeeding or bottle feeding, continue to do so on holiday. Even if your baby is coming up to an age where you might think of introducing solids, don't do so just before you go or when you're actually there. One change at a time is enough for your baby anyway – and weaning onto solids makes life that much more complicated for you.

If you are holidaying somewhere hot, your baby may need extra fluids. This might mean extra breastfeeds or if you're bottle feeding, or your baby's on mixed feeding, extra non-milk drinks. Take your baby's usual formula with you, and a few favourite pre-packed baby foods. Unless you're going somewhere really remote, commercial baby foods are available in chemists and supermarkets abroad. If you've the least reason to suspect the plumbing in your holiday home, then boil and cool the WATER before giving it to your baby, even if you've stopped doing that at home. Alternatively, offer non-carbonated mineral water but ask before buying if the brand you choose is suitable for a baby. Tummy upsets are bad enough at home but on holiday, away from your usual sources of advice, they can be really worrying. Try to keep your baby's diet basically unchanged. You may like to sample the local cuisine, and why not? But your baby might react to food he's not accustomed to. Even mothers in countries where spicy, oily foods are the norm tend to keep their babies on plainer, simpler fare at first.

See also TRAVEL

HONEY

Honey is a useful sweetener when you want to avoid sugar. However, there was a scare recently when some small babies contracted botulism after eating honey, and although this is rare, it would seem sensible to delay its introduction. One expert says honey should not be given until the age of 10 months.

HOSPITAL

Fortunately, hospital postnatal wards have almost all abandoned rigid feeding policies. This works in favour of breastfeeding, which rarely gets off to a good start under an old-fashioned '10 minutes a side, every four hours, no night feeds' regime. But – and it's a big 'but' – in practice, mothers are still given conflicting advice about breastfeeding. You may be 'allowed' to breastfeed on demand (see DEMAND FEEDING), but many women still report that they're told that this means 'no more often than every three hours'. Babies are often given unnecessary water (with dextrose or glucose), and even complementary bottles of formula milk (see also COMPLEMENTARY AND SUPPLEMENTARY BOTTLES). If you feed frequently, eyebrows are raised ('Not feeding again, Mrs X?'); babies are labelled 'greedy' if they need feeding often, or the mum is told 'Your baby's a little actress – she can't really need feeding'. Precious little help is available to those women who need help in getting the baby latched on (see LATCHING ON), or who develop problems. Breastfeeding mothers are still given free samples of formula to go home with, which we *know* works against breastfeeding, and which is in direct contravention of the code of practice on formula milk marketing (see WHO CODE). I could go on.

Of course, not all hospitals are like this. Hats off to those who have truly informed midwives, called lactation sisters, lactation consultants or whatever, able to devote time to breastfeeding mothers, because breastfeeding is recognised as important enough to have a member of staff whose main job it is to promote and help it. The lactation sister is instrumental in formulating ward policy, and acts as a watchdog to prevent the conflicting advice which can come with each change of shift with their pet theories on breastfeeding (some of those pet theories may actually work – but we should be basing hospital practice on sound research as well as practical knowledge. Anything else leads to a hotch-potch of opinions – with the poor mother losing out!). If you find it's difficult to breastfeed, you're not getting the help you'd like or that hospital policy works against you, then ask to speak to the ward sister. She may help you herself, or get someone who she knows is keen on and knowledgeable about breastfeeding to help you. It may well be that the advice you've received goes against ward policy on breastfeeding and the sister needs to know. If she can't help you, then don't get too anxious. Being informed and motivated yourself is a great plus point, and once you're home you'll be able to work things out differently. If you know, or even suspect, that babies in the hospital you're in get given bottles without the mothers' permission, then you can make sure that your baby is with you all the time *and* you can stick a note on the crib saying 'breast milk only, please'.

If you find yourself having to go into hospital while your baby is still being breastfed, then it may well be possible for your baby to be in with you, or else brought to you outside normal visiting hours for feeds. Similarly, if your baby needs to be hospitalised for any reason, of course you should be with him as much as you can, and that applies whether or not you're breastfeeding. If you are, then the health benefits of breastfeeding your baby when he's ill are very great.

HYGIENE

Young babies don't have a high resistance to infection at first although breastfeeding passes on ANTIBODIES that help to fight it in the first months. Hygiene is important however you feed, though you don't need to wash your breasts before feeding (people are still advised to do this, quite unnecessarily).

If you're BOTTLE FEEDING, you should be careful to sterilise all your baby's feeding equipment every time you use it (see STERILISING). This is essential for the first six months. Thereafter, it's probably not so vital as your baby will have built up a resistance to bacteria. Ideally, you should still keep up the routine if your baby has milk from a bottle, because bugs multiply so rapidly in warmed milk and because an older baby may hold his bottle himself, and it's then easier for it to be left lying around.

Normal washing in hot water with detergent followed by rinsing, will be enough to keep your baby's plates and spoons clean (there are no awkward corners, unlike bottles and teats, that can harbour germs). If you are giving solid food to a baby under four or five months, however, then it would be safest to sterilise, especially if the baby is bottle fed. Keep spouted cups clean by poking round the inside of the spout and the rim with a matchstick before washing carefully and rinsing (if you use milk in these cups, then sterilise at least occasionally). When your baby is having proper meals, you can start the habit of washing his hands before he eats. This is especially important if you have pets who may come into contact with your baby. If you have food or milk in the fridge, make sure you keep it covered, and discard it if it's not used within 48 hours. Don't keep made-up formula milk in the fridge for more than a day at a time.

HYPERACTIVITY

Hyperactivity is a diagnosis which may be applied to some children who are aggressive, sleepless, disruptive and with possible food allergies (see ALLERGY). It is not applicable to an energetic, lively child who also wakes at night a lot, and I don't think it's ever really applicable to babies under a year, either, although the parents of hyperactive children do often recall the sleepless nights, colicky screaming and apparent tummy pains of their child's babyhood. I feel that there is a deal of evidence pointing to dietary causes and FOOD INTOLERANCE in some cases of hyperactivity. It therefore makes sense to breastfeed exclusively, wean gradually and encourage a wholesome diet in your children, in an attempt to avoid this sort of allergic response.

See also ADDITIVES AND COLOURINGS

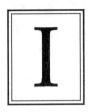

I

ICE CREAM*

Ice cream is not usually very suitable for babies, because when it is commercially made it is very sweet and high in fat and often has additives which you may prefer to avoid (though a little bit as an occasional treat isn't going to hurt him if your baby's diet already includes cow's milk). Try home-made ice cream instead; you can't avoid it being fatty but you can cut down on the sugar and avoid the additives.

ILLNESS

When your baby's ill you may wonder what to feed him on, if anything. Ask your doctor's advice about what to do in your particular circumstances. Generally speaking, babies do need to maintain their fluid intake when they're ill (see DEHYDRATION; DRINKS), and a loss of appetite for solid food is normal and, in fact, it's one of the symptoms of being ill or 'off colour'. If you're breastfeeding then carry on, and breastfeed as often as your baby will take it. Breast milk contains ANTIBODIES, it is easily digested and it gives security and comfort to an ill child. Even if your baby is on solids and well established on three meals a day and only the occasional feed, allow him to suck as often as he wants to. Your milk supply will build up quickly in response to these new demands. Bottle fed babies, and babies no longer on breast milk at all, are usually given 'half-strength feeds' – formula milk made up with twice the usual quantity of water, or ordinary full-fat pasteurised milk diluted with the same amount of water again. This is because of the very different composition of these milks compared to breast milk.

IMMUNITY

The healthy human body has a complex and highly efficient immune system, that recognises and fights invading diseases. Breastfeeding supports and develops the baby's immune system which is still incomplete at birth. Its ANTIBODIES protect the baby from a range of diseases, and it provides an important substance called immunoglobulin A (IgA) which protects against future ALLERGY.

INTRODUCTION TO SOLIDS

See WEANING

INVERTED NIPPLES

See NIPPLES

IRON

Iron is an element present in certain foods that's essential to health. Babies are born with iron stored in their bodies and it used to be thought that these stores run out after about six months, and so solids are then needed to supply it. It's now known that breast milk or formula milk supply iron to the baby, and that the iron from breast milk is especially easily absorbed. This means that the baby who is still on breast milk at six months and over should not be at risk of becoming anaemic. But if you have any worries about this, and your baby is slow to take to solid food that might supply him with iron, your doctor can run a quick and simple blood test to detect anaemia (lack of iron). Babies who are bottle fed may well be better off remaining on formula milk instead of going on to ordinary full-fat pasteurised milk at six months or over, unless they are on a good range of solids, including iron-rich foods. This is because it is poor in iron, and it is thought by some paediatricians to lead to iron-deficiency anaemia in babies who don't have a wide variety of solid foods as well as their milk. Foods that contain iron include vegetables, fruit, liver, kidneys, whole grains and red meat.

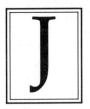

JAMS AND SPREADS

If you're keen for your baby to avoid unnecessary sugar, choose jams without it. Don't go for the ones with artificial sweeteners, such as sorbitol or saccharin, instead (that means avoiding the sorts marketed for diabetics). You can choose from a number of 'sugar-free' brands, or buy pear and apple spread which is available in health and wholefood shops. Your baby can have jam on his bread or toast as soon as you're sure he can cope. You can also use a spoonful of jam to flavour yoghurt or custard.

Savoury spreads with salt in them, such as Marmite, should be used very sparingly indeed, and again, wait for your baby to get used to bread first. Fortunately, you don't need much to get a good flavour. Try tahina (sesame seed paste) as a change. Spreads like fish or meat paste in jars aren't usually suitable for babies as they have ADDITIVES AND COLOURINGS in them. Those that don't should be fine, but again, use sparingly as they are likely to have a lot of salt in them, and keep in the fridge.

When? After your baby's used to BREAD.

JAUNDICE

Some babies, especially pre-term babies, are jaundiced in the first days of life. The skin of white babies looks yellow or tanned, and jaundiced babies of all ethnic groups may have a marked yellow tinge to the whites of the eyes. The jaundice is caused in most cases by a temporary inability of the liver to clear the blood of bilirubin, a substance produced when red blood cells are broken down. The bilirubin builds up and it is this that causes the yellow coloration. There is usually no need for treatment unless the level of bilirubin is high or persistent, if it appears the jaundice is caused by an infection or a blood group incompatibility with the mother (such as in Rhesus disease). A jaundiced baby may be sleepy and apathetic about feeding, so you may need to wake her for feeds. She may then drop off for a further snooze after no more than a minute at the breast (see SLEEPY BABY). There is no evidence that extra water helps a breastfed jaundiced baby as is often suggested. If you're breastfeeding, giving water to your baby could interfere with your MILK SUPPLY. Simply feed your baby often, as a good milk supply will be better for him than water. The extra fluid may help a bottle fed baby on formula milk however.

Another form of jaundice, known as breast milk jaundice, is very rare. It's thought to be caused by a substance in the breast milk interfering with liver function. You may be advised to take your baby off the breast for a short time, to allow the bilirubin level to fall and also to establish if it is in fact breast milk that's causing the jaundice (you should be EXPRESSING BREAST MILK in the meantime to keep up your supply). There's no reason why you can't continue to breastfeed after this, as long as your baby's jaundice is monitored so he can come off the breast milk again for a period, if it proves necessary.

JELLIES*

You can make fresh fruit jellies easily with juice or puréed fruit and gelatine. Babies like them, and they're a pleasant, healthy dessert. Commercial jellies are not really much more convenient, and they aren't as nutritious: they're often full of sugar and may contain additives and colourings.

When? From the time your baby has become used to the fruit used in the jelly (see WEANING).

JUICE

Babies don't need juice until they are taking foods other than milk. Yet orange juice is often suggested for babies as a supplement to either breast or formula milk. Oranges are known to be a food that often cause ALLERGY in people and so delaying it until at least six months is sensible. If a baby under this age seems

115

thirsty, then give him breast milk or water. If he spits the water out, then he can't be thirsty! If you want to give juice before the age when you start on mixed feeding, then apple juice would be a better choice. When you do give your baby juice to drink, it's best if it's unsweetened and well-diluted with water. This isn't because juice is harmful in any way, but because we know it's best to avoid foods and drinks which contain a lot of SUGAR, and because strongly-flavoured juice will be unpleasant to drink and if it's not well-diluted, it may be acidic and very high in calories.

Juice can be freshly-squeezed from the fruit or from a carton. Make sure you're buying pure fruit juice and not the stuff in similar looking packaging, which will be labelled not as 'fruit juice' but as 'fruit drink'. A look at the label will probably confirm that the ingredients contain water, sugar and possibly other things as well. Vegetable juices are available in cartons too, and you could offer your baby carrot juice, for example (again well-diluted).

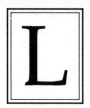

LABELS

I often say in this book that you should read the labels of pre-packaged foods. That way, at least you know something of what you're giving your baby to eat. I know that there's a lobby that points out that food-labelling isn't fully informative, and that food manufacturers get away with a lot because regulations and codes of practice don't yet insist on the full story. However, in the meantime, you can learn something, and pre-packaged baby foods are usually well-labelled in comparison with other foods. Remember that foods are listed in descending order of quantity.

LACTATION

The production of milk by the breasts.
See BREASTFEEDING

LACTOSE

Lactose is the sugar present in milk, including breast milk. Some people are intolerant to milk because once they get beyond childhood, they do not produce enough of the enzyme lactase and this is needed to metabolise the lactose. The symptoms of lactose intolerance in infancy and childhood are DIARRHOEA and failure to thrive (see also FOOD INTOLERANCE). Interestingly, there is a school of thought that links COLIC in breastfed babies with lactose intolerance. Many babies take a very long breastfeed in the mornings. It could be that that long feed overloads the baby's tummy and the amount of lactose present is too much for the gut to cope with all in one go. As a result, about 12 hours later (at 'colic' time), the excess lactose has fermented

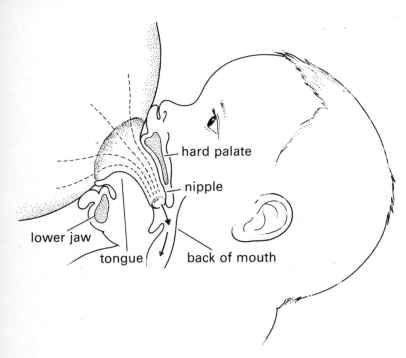

A baby latches on by opening his mouth wide and taking the nipple into his mouth so that the lower lip is turned back, his tongue is under the nipple and his mouth is centred on the nipple. This gives him a good chance to get the nipple well back into his mouth, and to shape it with his tongue and jaw.

and this causes WIND pains. Mothers have found a solution to colic by EXPRESSING BREAST MILK in the morning, as this slows down the flow, and the baby doesn't have to swallow more to keep up with the otherwise overwhelming amount of milk. Or else they find that feeding from only one side at a time throughout the day and not even offering the second breast, also has the effect of reducing the volume of milk going into the baby (you should only do this if you're confident of your milk supply, and of the fact that your baby's gaining weight adequately).

LAMB*

Lamb is a good first meat for a baby. Small lamb chops with the fat removed can be given as finger food but you do need to be careful that your baby doesn't snap off any shards of bone.

When? From the second stage of WEANING.

LATCHING ON

Your baby needs to latch on correctly to the breast in order to breastfeed well. The actual mechanisms of sucking are very complex, and work is still being done to establish what actually happens to the nipple, and to the baby's jaw, tongue and palate. We do know that the baby compresses the nipple with his tongue, pushing the nipple against the hard palate in waves, and this squeezes the milk out. In order for this to happen, you need to make sure your baby's latched on. Before you actually offer the breast to your baby, think about how you're holding him; make sure his body is turned towards you, with his head slightly tilted back – a common mistake is to have the baby on his back, expecting him to turn his head through 45 degrees. New babies – and new mothers – might need a lot of help in getting this position right. You might need pillows to raise your baby up a little, and to support your arms.

If you have sore NIPPLES when you're breastfeeding, check your baby's latched on right, and check it, too, if your baby's not gaining WEIGHT well or seems to need feeding every hour for more than a day or so. Don't just assume he's 'on right' if it looks as though he has a lot of nipple and areola in his mouth. That might appear to be the case from your position above the baby, but underneath, it might be a different story. Many women have ended up with sore nipples because the baby is chewing on the end, with only the very tip of the nipple over the lower jaw. If your baby's not latched on correctly, take him off and try again. For some, this might mean a lot of time and patience at several feeds. For others, after the baby's done it right once, they never look back. The baby is rewarded with a comfortable, productive sucking position, and he adopts it every time from then on. An older baby, and a baby who has learnt how to feed well, can often

119

get himself latched on from whatever position he finds himself in. But in the early days especially, take care and get your feeding position looked at by a midwife if you have any doubts.
See also POSITION AT BREAST

LEAKING FROM BREASTS

This can vary from being non-existent, a minor irritation or it can be a major problem. Breasts that produce milk don't always hang on to their stores of it. If you produce a lot of milk, you're probably more likely to leak, involuntarily (see TOO MUCH MILK). The tiny muscles holding the milk respond to the pressure of a lot of milk too well, and open the gates to release it. Some women who have an efficient LET-DOWN REFLEX find that they even respond to a baby's cry (any baby's cry – not necessarily only their own!), or to thoughts of babies, by leaking. I know one mother who found she 'leaked' whenever she saw a particularly 'weepy' film! For others, the situation only arises occasionally when their baby unexpectedly goes for several hours between feeds or when they're feeding from one side, at which point the other side starts to release milk as well. Women who don't leak at all may have an especially good 'tone' in those muscles surrounding the milk cells, and they manage to hold everything in no matter what. However irritating leaking is, it is a problem that's at its worse in the first weeks of feeding. Thereafter, for most women, it settles down along with the whole process of lactation (see BREASTFEEDING). Practical measures to cope with it might help in the meantime if it doesn't get better on its own.

When leaking happens from the non-feeding side, press against that nipple with the heel of your hand or with your forearm. You can usually do this unobtrusively, without altering the position of the feeding baby. Breast pads will help with leaking between feeds; you can buy disposable ones, washable ones, or you can use pieces of cut-up towelling, towelling nappies, soft cotton hankies (men's hankies are best, because they're big enough to be folded into four and still remain a reasonable size) or a nappy liner. You wear the pad, or whatever you're using, inside your bra, and it absorbs the flow. You then discard the pad when it gets soggy. Dark clothing hides the wet patches best. A plastic cover for your mattress, or your side of it, protects against leaks at night.

LEEKS*

Wash leeks carefully to remove any traces of soil between the layers – the easiest way to do this is to slice them lengthways and then across, rinsing the pieces through in a colander. Boil or steam, then mash, sieve or purée.

When? From the first stage of WEANING.

LEFT-OVERS

Don't feel guilty if you sometimes save left-overs from your baby's meals, but there are a few do's and don'ts. Food starts to deteriorate as soon as it's cooked but not necessarily drastically or dangerously. If it's left long enough, however, bacteria will form and multiply, and make the food unsafe to eat, but keeping the food in the fridge will slow down this process for a period. For a baby, it's safe to keep cooked food in the fridge for 24 hours. Do put the food straight into the fridge and keep it covered. If you've been spoonfeeding your baby from a bowl and she doesn't finish it, don't put the bowl in the fridge for later use. This is because the saliva that's been on the spoon will have mixed with the food, and this will hasten the bacterial break-down. If you're not sure of how much food your baby will take at a sitting, then put only a little at a time into the serving bowl. You can then put the unserved, left-over food in the fridge. It's not safe to put your baby's bottle back in the fridge if she doesn't finish it as milk is especially likely to deteriorate and become harmful to your baby if left like this. Making up feeds in advance and storing them in the fridge for up to 24 hours is fine, though. When you come to serve the food again, you can serve it straight from the fridge unless it has meat in it. If it does, you must heat and boil it in order to destroy any harmful bacteria. It's safe to keep some food you've cooked for your baby to eat later along with food for yourself, as long as you refrigerate it straightaway, covered, and you boil anything containing meat before serving it.

121

LEMONS

See CITRUS FRUITS

LENTILS

See BEANS AND PULSES

LET-DOWN REFLEX

During breastfeeding, some of the milk you make lies in reservoirs behind the nipple, and it becomes available to your baby as soon as he starts to suck. The rest of the milk is stored in the lobes within the breast. The lobes are linked to the nipple by means of the milk ducts and the breast milk needs to be let down from the lobes, into the ducts and then into the nipple before the baby can receive it. For this to happen, and for the baby to have a satisfying feed, the let-down reflex has to work. This is caused by a hormonal reaction. When your baby sucks, the very action of his sucking produces a hormonal response in your body; the nerve endings in the nipple transmit messages to your brain, and the pituitary gland in the brain releases the hormone OXYTOCIN into the blood stream. Under the influence of the oxytocin, the tiny muscles which surround the milk cells in the lobes contract, squeezing the milk out and into the ducts. The milk comes out with some force at times. If your baby breaks off in the middle of a feed, you might notice that the milk continues to flow for some seconds – in a stream, not a trickle. In this way, the let-down reflex actually makes it easier for babies to feed. The baby at the breast needs to set the feed in motion, as it were, sucking and swallowing in turn. But once the let-down works, he has less need to suck continuously. He will have to swallow the milk as it flows into his mouth, and he will have to give the occasional suck, and maybe the occasional series of sucks, to maintain the let-down (in fact, there's more than one let-down a feed and there could be several). But if breastfeeding's going well, and you watch your baby at your breast, you'll see the suck-swallow-suck-swallow pattern change to a suck-swallow-swallow-swallow-suck-swallow-swallow etc. In bottle feeding, the baby has to maintain a consistent suck-swallow-suck pattern, to keep up the flow of milk through the teat.

Once breastfeeding's established the let-down works more or less straight away. It can even work in response to your baby's cry or totally unbidden (see also LEAKING FROM BREASTS). This is more likely in women who have fed one or more babies. It's an involuntary response so you can't will it to work or prevent it. You might feel a sort of tingling when it happens although some women never actually feel anything. At first, however, it can take a minute or two, or three, to get the let-down working. Restricting the length of breastfeeds makes no sense, when this is realised, as you could be restricting the time your baby has available to get the milk flowing. Let-down failure may happen to anyone at any time. Stress, depression or anxiety in the mother can all interfere with it – this may be part of the reason babies sometimes feed better if you're in a quiet place, where you feel more relaxed. Consistent let-down failure is more worrying as it will mean your baby is very often unsatisfied after a feed and may fail to gain WEIGHT. It could be caused by your baby LATCHING ON to the nipple incorrectly (see also POSITION AT BREAST). Or it could mean that you need to make a special effort to relax at feed times.

LETTUCE

Washed lettuce leaves, chopped to a suitable size, can be given to babies able to chew reasonably well.

When? From the time your baby can chew – about nine months.

LIMES

See CITRUS FRUITS

LIVER*

Liver's a good source of iron, as well as having the other nutritional qualities of meat. Lamb's liver is a good first meat, offered to your baby once he's used to first-stage fruit, vegetables and cereals. You may need to purée or mash it after cooking, at first, depending on how old your baby is. Otherwise chop it into suitable-sized pieces. Chicken liver is suitable for a baby, but pig's liver is likely to be too tough unless it's puréed. This is best delayed until nine months or a year in a baby who shows signs of FOOD INTOLERANCE.

When? Lamb's liver – from the second stage of WEANING; other livers – after your baby is used to lamb's liver.

LUNCH*

Lunch is normally one of the main meals once your baby's on three meals a day. It's up to you whether lunch or tea/supper is *the* main meal. It depends on what suits your family. Ideas for lunch for a baby established on second-stage feeding include: chopped liver, pasta and carrots; chicken, mashed potato and cauliflower; cheesy potato and peas; minced beef on toast, with chopped, cooked tomato. If you just have sandwiches at lunch-time, then your baby will be fine having a sandwich too. You can then eat your main meal together later on.

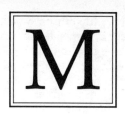

MANGO

Delicious, not too strong in flavour and easy to prepare, mango is a good first-stage weaning food. Cut in half lengthways and scoop out the flesh. Cook as you would an APPLE, at first, or simply put the amount you need into a food processor or blender and purée. Mango can be eaten as finger food, in slices or cubes, by an older baby able to chew.

When? From the first stage of WEANING.

MARGARINE

An alternative to butter, margarine is made from vegetable oil, or a blend of vegetable oils, mixed with other ingredients (such as whey, colorants, water and vitamin D). Current advice to people concerned about adopting a healthier diet is to use a polyunsaturated margarine (such as the ones made from sunflower oil) in preference to butter which is high in saturated fats. For a baby of under a year this is not crucial – what you spread on your baby's bread is going to be no more than a very small part of his diet unless you use, unwisely, vast quantities. However, if you are concerned about longer-term effects of his dietary likes and dislikes, it would be a good idea to use polyunsaturated margarine to get him used to it.

MASTITIS

Literally translated, this means inflammation of the breast. It doesn't necessarily mean there is an actual infection there. The symptoms of mastitis are similar to those for BLOCKED DUCTS. In fact, mastitis often starts with a blocked duct, and many doctors, especially, use the terms blocked duct and mastitis interchangeably. In fact, it can be difficult to say where a blocked duct ends and mastitis begins. If the lump you feel in your breast is tender or sore, and/or there is a red patch on the skin of the affected breast, then it's clear that the immune system has gone into action, and this inflammation is the response to the blockage. You may also feel hot and shivery just like an attack of flu. What happens is this; milk from the blocked duct(s) leaks into the blood stream in the breast because it is under pressure. The blood recognises the 'foreignness' of the milk, and starts to fight it. The result is the inflammation you can usually both see and feel. This sort of mastitis should be called, as some writers have done, non-infective mastitis, or obstructive mastitis; and it is by far the most common sort. However, it can become infective; the pressure on the milk ducts makes them wider, and bacteria can enter them more easily. This is why antibiotics from your doctor may be advisable and these will prevent the infection developing, and treat any infection that's already developed (see also MEDICATION AND BREAST MILK). *But* you should try to get rid of your mastitis with other measures as well and there may not be any need to use antibiotics in the first place. All the suggestions to be found under blocked ducts are worth trying, either before you use the antibiotics or in addition to using them. Whatever you do, don't stop feeding (see below). This will make the problem worse, and you could even end up with a BREAST ABSCESS. If it's painful to feed, try putting a hot water bottle wrapped in a towel against the sore area, although I accept this may be difficult to manoeuvre when the baby has to be fitted in as well. Gentle massage followed by gentle expressing will help, too (see EXPRESSING BREAST MILK).

Infective mastitis has similar symptoms to obstructive mastitis, though the pain may be more acute and you may feel worse generally. The infection is caused by bacteria entering the breast via the nipple, sometimes from a germ in the baby's nose, or from a cracked nipple that's failed to heal up properly. The treatment is the same as described above.

Some doctors advise stopping feeding during a bout of mastitis, or expressing and then discarding the milk. Stopping feeding is the worst thing you can do and many women cannot express their milk nearly as efficiently as a feeding baby can do it for them!

They say this because there is an idea that the milk may be harmful to the baby. There is no justification for this view. Even if you have an infection, as opposed to an inflammation, and the infection reaches your milk, your baby will already have been exposed to the bacteria causing the infection. It would make sense to continue feeding, as your breast milk will contain the ANTIBODIES needed to fight the infection. Some women are unlucky enough to get repeated attacks of mastitis and it's worth thinking why this should be. It might be caused by some infection in your baby's nose that never quite clears up (in which case, he'll need treating as well as you). You may be producing TOO MUCH MILK, or wearing a bra that is too tight. Check, too, that when you hold your baby you aren't putting pressure on your breast with your arm, hand or fingers. Stress may also be a factor, and you may need to make a conscious effort to simplify your life to cope with it, if that's possible.

MEAT*

It's certainly possible for children to grow up healthily without meat (see VEGETARIANISM) but in this society, most babies are from meat-eating families. In our diets, meat plays an important part in supplying protein, fat, vitamins and minerals. Fresh or frozen meat is best for your baby. Meat pastes, spreads, cured or prepared meat (like beefburgers, bacon, ready-crumbed chicken and so on) may contain SALT, flavourings, ADDITIVES AND COLOURINGS that your baby would be better off without.

Your baby's first solids will be certain fruit, vegetables and cereals. You can offer meat as a second-stage weaning food, once he's used to those other items. LAMB is an excellent first choice as it is not one of the meats most associated with FOOD INTOLERANCE, and it has a mild, pleasant flavour that babies like. The next meat your baby can move on to could be BEEF, followed by veal, CHICKEN and then pork. You can also give your baby OFFAL, and, as much of this cooks quickly, it can be a convenient, easy meal. If you can get it, 'organic' meat, from animals which have been reared naturally and without the use of intensive farming methods, is likely to be better for your baby, and you. Some butchers do sell this sort of meat, and

127

some supermarkets have started selling chickens that have been raised naturally, too.

You can cook meat for your baby in the same ways as you'd cook it for yourself. You can purée most sorts of meat if you have a blender or food processor, or chop it up and offer it as finger food. Cut off the fat, or as much of it as you can, and try not to use a lot of fat in cooking. Too much fat could be indigestible for a small tummy.

When? From the second stage of WEANING, starting with lamb, and moving on to beef, veal, chicken and pork.

MEDICATION AND BREAST MILK

This is a medical question and outside the scope of this book. The two points to remember are that virtually all drugs of whatever sort (and I'm including medication and illegal and legal drugs in this), do get into the BREAST MILK, just as they reach your bloodstream. Sometimes this matters a lot, sometimes it may not be important. It depends on the drug, on the amount the mother is taking, how long she needs to take it for, the weight of the baby and the strength of her need for the drug. If you need medication for some reason, tell the doctor you're breastfeeding so he can offer you an alternative, possibly more suitable drug. NCT breastfeeding counsellors have access to expert knowledge and up-to-date pharmacological information on the effects of drugs in breast milk, so if your doctor's unsure, or unable to reassure you, you can try this avenue for more details (see HELP AND ADVICE).

Nicotine depresses the milk supply, and gets into the milk. This means breastfeeding mothers should give up SMOKING, although this is not a reason for switching to the bottle if you really can't give up. Try cutting down, at least. ALCOHOL gets through too. Illegal drugs – whether 'soft' like cannabis or 'hard' like heroin – also get to the baby via breast milk. If you habitually take any drug, then you need to discuss the issue of breastfeeding with someone who knows the extent of your problem before you decide on a feeding method. The same applies to mothers who are taking constant medication to control conditions like epilepsy and asthma.

See also CHEMICALS AND BREAST MILK; CONTRACEPTION

MELON

Melon is refreshing and easy to prepare. Don't cook it, a baby just starting on solids should be able to manage it, as long as you mash it up finely. An older baby will be able to enjoy melon as finger food, if you choose a firmer variety that can be sliced. Try mixing melon in with natural yoghurt, to flavour it.

When? From the first stage of WEANING.

MENSTRUATION

You'll almost certainly find your periods cease for some time when you breastfeed. When they return, it's possible your baby may 'go off' the breast for some reason (see BREAST REFUSAL). It could be that the breast milk tastes slightly different. Usually, a baby who does this returns to the breast when the period is finishing. See also CONTRACEPTION

METABOLIC DISORDERS

Metabolic disorders are conditions that affect the digestive process, and hence the way the body's nourished. They include disorders such as diabetes, COELIAC DISEASE, PKU, PYLORIC STENOSIS, and some forms of FOOD INTOLERANCE. Control of the diet can usually help to mitigate their effects. There's a body of evidence which strongly suggests that in many cases, the risk of non-congenital disorders (that is, the baby isn't born with them) can be reduced by exclusive breastfeeding for at least the first four to six months of life or that the severity of disorders can be mitigated. The introduction of foods or fluids other than breast milk can so alter the environment of the gut that the baby's susceptibility to metabolic disturbance is increased.
See USEFUL ADDRESSES

MICROWAVE COOKING

Microwave ovens cook food from the inside out. Although there has been some controversy about whether microwaves damage

129

the food molecules, there is little real evidence that microwaving is any more detrimental to food than conventional cooking. I can't see any reason why food for your baby should not be prepared in this way. However, there are some 'don'ts' when it comes to baby's bottles of milk. You cannot sterilise adequately in a microwave. And to use it to heat a baby's feed is unsafe, too, because the way the microwave heats means that the bottle itself is cooler than the milk inside. It is therefore easy to give a baby a dangerously scalding hot feed from a bottle which has merely felt warm to the touch.

MIDWIFE

See HELP AND ADVICE

MILK

All mammals produce milk to nourish their young, and over the millenia, the milk of each species has evolved in such a way that it's custom-made to fit the growth pattern and food needs of the baby otter . . . calf . . . chimp . . . dolphin . . . human! Milk isn't essential for us or any other mammal beyond infancy, but because COW'S MILK, in particular, is such a convenient and cheap source of nutrients for us here in the West, we drink a lot of it, as babies, children and as adults.

BREAST MILK is best for your baby in the first year. If you need or want to use a substitute, then you should use a modified baby FORMULA MILK. Ordinary, full-fat pasteurised cow's milk is safe for most babies from about six months although at first it should be boiled and diluted. It is not ideal as a major source of nourishment at this age, however. Formula milk is better because it supplies the nutrients your baby still needs, in a form better suited to his digestion. If your baby is intolerant to cow's milk – and it's been estimated that about 10 per cent of infants are – and you don't want to change from bottle to breast (see CHANGING: FROM BOTTLE TO BREAST), then your doctor may advise a formula based on SOYA MILK. GOAT'S MILK isn't normally considered suitable for infants.

You don't actually need to drink milk yourself when you're breastfeeding though I still hear people who should know better say you need to drink it in order to make it. Milk is an excellent source of protein and calcium in particular, and if you like it, then go ahead. Some experts have suggested that if you drink a lot of it you may just be increasing the chances of your baby becoming intolerant to cow's milk, as his system won't be able to cope with more than the merest trace of cow's milk protein in your breast milk. There's no proof of this as yet, though the evidence is strong enough to suggest that there is no point in deliberately increasing your milk intake, and so keeping it within the limits of what you would normally drink anyway is the most sensible policy. If your baby cries or seems to have COLIC, cutting down on, or cutting out, DAIRY PRODUCTS, especially milk, is worth a try (see FOOD INTOLERANCE).

If your baby starts to go off milk at some time towards the end of his first year – and some do, whether breast or bottle fed – then ask your doctor's advice. Your baby may accept milk in a cup, or mixed with other foods. It's possible to make sure he gets enough of the right sorts of nutrients by paying attention to other parts of his diet, but you may need special help from a dietician to ensure this.

MILK BANK

A milk bank is a unit where human breast milk is stored for babies whose mothers are unable or unwilling to breastfeed, or to supplement the milk of mothers who aren't producing it in sufficient quantities. In most cases, banked human milk is used for a PRE-TERM BABY or a sick baby in the hospital special care unit. It's donated by mothers who express their milk for this purpose. Different banks have different policies on what they then do, the milk can be pooled and then pasteurised, or otherwise heat-treated to kill bacteria.

Recently, fear of AIDS has led to the closure of milk banks. This is because the virus thought to cause Aids has been found in breast milk, and one or two babies are thought to have contracted Aids via their mothers' milk. Although pasteurisation has been shown to kill the virus, and samples of milk could be tested both before and after treatment and before and after pooling, health authorities have decided to save a few pounds and close the milk banks. Aids is a huge problem, of course, and it would be tragic to risk any transmission of the virus, but wholesale closure of milk banks looks not so much like an over-reaction to a situation that could be dealt with by relatively small changes, as an excuse to save money and hassle. It's probably easier to feed pre-term babies on formula milk, which doesn't need to be specially collected, treated and stored by the hospital (though it has to be said that the collecting was often done by volunteers, such as NCT women who organised local 'milk runs'), and all the testing is done by the milk companies. Result? Fewer headaches for the hospital, and no lingering worries about Aids scares, ill-founded though they are. One might regard the loss of milk banks with greater tolerance if there was evidence that more women were being helped to feed their pre-term babies on their own breast milk, and that special care staff and training are to be increased for this to happen . . .

MILK SUPPLY

The most common reason why women give up breastfeeding is because they have worries about their milk supply. Basically, they feel they don't have enough to either keep the baby happy or keep him growing. In almost all cases correct action leads to an increase in the milk supply. To get your milk supply going, feed your newborn baby frequently. This means as often as he wants, and more often if your breasts are full and uncomfortable, or if he sleeps more than three hours between feeds (see DEMAND FEEDING). If you think you may be short of milk, then feed your baby more often. This will stimulate your breasts to produce more milk. Introducing COMPLEMENTARY AND SUP-PLEMENTARY BOTTLES of formula milk will *decrease* your milk supply, not increase it. If you have already given formula, and you still want to increase your breast milk supply so you can drop these 'comps', then you need to consider cutting out the formula altogether, so your baby can satisfy all his feeding and sucking needs at the breast, and not at a teat. Dropping all the 'comps' in one go may be difficult if you have been giving several; your milk supply won't increase immediately, and you'll have one cross and hungry baby. Instead, do it gradually, by reducing the 'comps' by one every few days, or by offering only half the usual amount of formua (see CHANGING: FROM BOTTLE TO BREAST). This will mean your baby will be hungry sooner, and more ready to suck from the breast. Check your baby's position on the breast (see LATCHING ON; POSITION AT BREAST), or get someone informed about breastfeeding to do it for you. She may not be able to stimulate a good supply if she's not well fixed. Think about whether your baby is at the breast long enough. If you're deliberately switching her to the second side in order to fit in both breasts at each feed, she may not have had time to receive as much calorie-rich HIND MILK to gain weight satisfactorily. On the other hand, some babies gain more weight feeding little and often, being switched from one breast to another and back again at each feed. This seems to encourage a series of let-down reflexes, and this therefore gets more milk into the baby (see LET-DOWN REFLEX). If you've been following one regime without success, then try the other. Try to encourage your baby to get his sucking comfort from you and not from a dummy. Either reduce his time with the dummy or if you can, cut it out altogether. Don't give water or juice either.

Also pay attention to your diet, eat nourishing snacks throughout the day and don't try to lose weight with a reducing diet (see DIET AND BREASTFEEDING). Rest – even bedrest for a couple of days – will help too. And give yourself a week for consciously increasing your supply. Some mothers find that they can then relax a bit, as the supply has caught up with baby's needs and they only need to feed as often as the baby wants. Others find they need to keep up the regime for longer.

However, do consider whether you really have cause to worry about your milk supply. Some babies do gain WEIGHT slowly, quite naturally, and some healthy babies take as much as three weeks or more to regain their birthweight (though if a baby is as slow as this to regain its birthweight, it would be sensible to make special efforts to ensure a good milk supply by adopting the measurements suggested above). The occasional week when your baby gains little or nothing is no cause for anxiety as long as his general weight is going up well enough. If your baby is gaining weight well, has plenty of dirty or wet nappies each day (say around six) and seems to be healthy and thriving, then you have enough milk. Plenty of babies fit this description and they still make their mothers think they are hungry at least some of the time. For instance, if your baby doesn't 'settle' between every feed, yes, that may mean he is a bit hungry still. It may mean other things as well, of course – about 100 other things! Offer him the breast again even if you feel 'there's nothing there'. Chances are there'll be something, and your baby may get comfort from being on the breast anyway. Never think 'he's had X minutes each side and he's still hungry – he needs a bottle'. X minutes a side may be less than he needs at that particular time; he may need to be on for longer in order to increase your milk supply anyway for next time!

Decreasing your milk supply can be done, too, and when your baby's on solids, it usually happens gradually and naturally, because the breasts don't get the same stimulation (see also TOO MUCH MILK). However, whereas in the early weeks of breast-feeding infrequent feeding almost always leads to the milk supply disappearing, a mother feeding an older baby only once or twice a day is usually able to keep up her milk indefinitely. And if she ever needs to increase her milk very quickly, for instance if her baby's ill and needs extra breast milk, then this is usually very easy. It's in the first few months that you may need to really work at increasing your milk supply, when there seems to be a gap between what you produce and what your baby needs.

MINCE*

Mince is the same as minced meat and although the mince you buy ready-made from the butcher is usually beef, you can mince any meat yourself or ask your butcher to do it for you. It's a good way to introduce your baby to MEAT. If you can afford to have a choice, don't buy the cheapo-cheapo minced beef that's barely a pale pink in colour. It's very high in FAT, and for a baby very fatty food is hard to digest. Buy the more expensive sort, sometimes billed 'best mince' or 'minced steak', or else buy stewing or braising steak and mince it yourself. Because it's ground up into small pieces, mince is quicker to cook than other cuts of meat. Cook it on the stove top, in its own fat, without adding any more to the pan. When it's browned, the fat will start to run out. You can then drain the fat, add just enough water to cover the mince and continue cooking up to boiling point. Then lower the heat, put a lid on the pan and simmer until the meat is tender (ten to 20 minutes depending on the quantity of mince).

When? From the second stage of WEANING.

MINERALS

Minerals are inorganic substances, present in food, and essential to growth and health. A list of examples would include calcium, potassium, zinc and iron. In infancy, your child will need certain minerals, but at a much lower level than he requires later on. Too high a mineral load could overwork his kidneys and lead to serious illness (see SALT). This is why cow's milk needs its mineral level artificially adjusting as part of the process of modifying it, in order to make formula milk.

MIXED FEEDING

Mixed feeding is a term used to describe the stage when a baby's major source of nourishment is still milk, while being given increasing amounts of solid food.
See WEANING

MONTGOMERY'S TUBERCLES

Montgomery's tubercles are the tiny exit points of glands on your nipple and areola. You can see them as little spots, maybe a dozen or so on each breast, and they appear at the very start of pregnancy. The glands secrete a small amount of lubricating fluid that softens your nipples, and which kills surface bacteria, keeping your nipples clean and preparing them for breastfeeding, although don't confuse this fluid with COLOSTRUM. The tubercles and glands function during breastfeeding itself as well.

MUESLI*

Muesli is a mixture of cereals, fruit and nuts that you can buy pre-packaged or make yourself from the ingredients of your choice. It's usually eaten for breakfast, with milk. You can give your baby muesli as long as you know she can cope with all or most of the ingredients separately. Muesli could be her first introduction to NUTS if she is already used to the cereal in the muesli and the fruit (nuts must be ground, however). The best sort of muesli for her is free of sugar, and ground up finely. You can grind the mixture in a blender or food processor if it has large lumps in it, or chunks of nut. Bought baby muesli is available but you need to check it's not too sweet. It may be sugar-free according to the label, but contain lashings of sweeteners such as honey or maltose. Don't forget, if you want your baby to avoid COW'S MILK until he's older because of the risk of FOOD INTOLERANCE, you can give muesli made with water, formula milk or by EXPRESSING BREAST MILK.

When? From the second stage of WEANING, when your baby is able to cope with cereal and fruit.

MUSHROOMS

Wash mushrooms well before you cook them for your baby, and trim the very end of the stalk. Peeling them removes some of the nutrients so don't do it. Chop the mushrooms and boil in a small amount of water, simmering until tender. You can mash or purée them. Older babies who can chew can have larger pieces of cooked mushroom as finger food. Uncooked mushroom may be fine towards the end of the first year, as long as it's cut up finely. In fact mushrooms are often among the foods commonly disliked by babies and children – perhaps it's an acquired taste.

When? From the second stage of WEANING. As finger food: from about eight months.

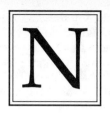

NECTARINES

See PEACHES AND NECTARINES

NIGHT FEEDS

Almost all babies need feeding during the night at first as they make no distinction between day-time and night-time, although some seem to start reacting to some sort of difference within the first week or two. Night feeds are important if you're breastfeeding. Your breast milk supply needs stimulating round the clock in order to establish the whole process.

Make night feeds easier on yourself by keeping them low-key. This will help your baby go back to sleep again more quickly. Don't allow your baby to work herself up into a frenzy of hunger, and try to feed her soon after she wakes. It's a matter of your own preference whether you have your baby in the same room (and/or the same bed) as you. My own personal preference is to have the baby in the same room until the age of six months or so, at which time the baby is too big for a crib and able to go into the 'big' cot. That way, you're on hand to wake up as soon as the baby cries and you can feed her in your bed, without crossing a cold landing in the dark, while his cries get louder and wake everybody else including the neighbours! On the other hand, you may not be able to relax enough to go to sleep if your baby's in the same room, while you listen for the tiniest movement and the faintest squeak. Banish all ideas that you're somehow 'spoiling' a baby by having him in the same room, by the way. I've heard people say the baby 'has to get used to being on his own'. That's true, I suppose, but you have a whole childhood ahead to teach him that! The first few months of a baby's life shouldn't be dogged with the pressures of discipline. Another way of keeping the feeds low-key is to feed in the dark, or with just the glow of a night light or low watt bulb to help you. You'll need to change your baby's nappy each time at first as it will probably be soaking. As she gets older, though, she will urinate less frequently, and you should be able to leave her in the same nappy, especially if you put her in a double nappy (if you use terries), or in a thicker, more absorbent disposable. You should, of course, still change her if she has nappy rash, or if she has passed a large bowel motion. Take her into bed with you to feed, and practice lying down, or at least reclining, while feeding (see POSITION AT BREAST). At least, you will get some sleep this way. It doesn't matter if you drop off and wake up ages later, with your baby still in your arms. In fact, some of the most pleasant memories of babyhood may turn out to be those close, quiet times, snuggled down with a little person next to you!

If you're bottle feeding, you could take up a kettle, formula milk and bottle to make up a feed when your baby wakes. This is better than taking up the ready-made bottle which might mean the milk is hanging round for hours in a warmish room. The easiest option may be to go down and fetch a bottle from the fridge, warming it by standing it in a jug of hot water. You could be well-prepared and have the water ready warmed in a thermos to save boiling the kettle.

Many babies still wake up for feeds at the age of three or four months although if it's more than twice a night, every night, it would be reasonable to work out ways of reducing the demand. Some families who all share the same bed – and it happens these days, just as it used to happen with previous generations and as it still happens in other societies round the world – find they don't really mind the baby waking up frequently in the night. In fact, it becomes a non-event. The baby learns to 'help herself' to the breast, and the mother barely wakes. If this isn't for you, you can think of other solutions. Could you, for instance, wake your baby when you go to bed, so you are only woken once or twice? This strategy can be tried a lot sooner than three to four months, of course. Don't play with your baby or let him 'socialise' with you, settle him with a feed by all means and then put him back in his crib or cot. Ideally, babies older than four to six months who are bottle fed should do without full bottles in the night – it's so easy to overfeed them this way. This isn't a worry with breast milk as the baby is likely to regulate his own appetite better. However, neither breast or bottle fed babies actually need milk in the night at this age if they are healthy and gaining weight well. They are waking, as everyone does for short times throughout the night, but they're unable to get to sleep again without the comfort of sucking. You could think about introducing a dummy although this can be difficult. A bottle fed baby could have WATER instead, or his milk could be very gradually watered down. Don't feel unusual if you find it's easier just to give in and offer the breast, or a bottle of water or formula. Plenty of babies wake up in the night during the first year. It's often easier to change sleeping habits beyond this age, when your child starts to understand language, when his memory allows him to remember that you're never very far away, and when he may gradually lose interest in the breast or bottle as a matter of course.

NIPPLES

Nipples, like breasts, come in a variety of forms, and not everyone has the perfectly circular and pointing nipples that you see on topless models. Some are very large in comparison to others, but this doesn't seem to make much difference to the establishment of breastfeeding. But, you may need to take your nipples into account when positioning your baby at the breast. For example, a few women have nipples whose tips are slightly off-centre, and the baby's position needs to be adjusted accordingly. The tip of the nipple needs to be centred in the baby's mouth, even if that makes the baby asymmetrical in relation to the rest of the nipple (see LATCHING ON; POSITION AT BREAST).

The nipple and surrounding areola are among the most sensitive parts of the female body. They are richly supplied with nerve endings that transmit sensations to the brain, and this is important in breastfeeding as it's these sensations that spark off the LET-DOWN REFLEX. Each nipple has tiny glands which supply a fluid to protect and soften it during pregnancy and lactation. The exit point of these glands are called MONTGOMERY'S TUBERCLES and they look like little spots. Each nipple has about 20 little openings that allow the milk to go into the baby's mouth. Each one is connected to a milk duct (some ducts may converge

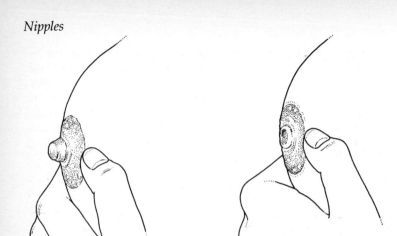

A normal nipple protrudes if the areola is pinched.
An inverted nipple retracts if the areola is pinched.

before they get to the nipple, so you may have more ducts than openings).

Flat nipples   Lots of women appear to have flat nipples that seem to be no more than a very slightly bumpy spot of colour on the end of their breasts! Or you may have one nipple that seems flatter than the other one. It's sometimes thought that flat nipples are bound to make breastfeeding very difficult, but this needn't be the case. Flat nipples are almost always protractile, so they stand out under stimulation by the cold or by touch and in many cases, this ability to stand out improves as pregnancy progresses, and later, as breastfeeding gets underway. They need to stand out, as the baby needs something to latch on to and to draw into the back of his mouth.

If your nipples aren't protractile in pregnancy, then you can help to improve them by gentle rolling (either by yourself or with your partner) between finger and thumb. Alternatively, try the technique outlined for inverted nipples. Flat nipples may not be a serious difficulty in themselves, but they can make it even more important to be careful about position. ENGORGEMENT has the effect of making flat nipples even flatter, and correct positioning more difficult (see POSITION AT BREAST). A baby who's sleepy or unwilling to suck won't be helped by nipples that only stand out a bit. Dealing with the engorgement is essential, and you can also be helped by stimulating your nipples or shaping them with your finger and thumb before putting your baby to the breast. Some women have found wearing BREAST SHELLS for short periods of time before they expect to feed their babies is helpful – the shell draws the nipple out into a better shape.

Inverted nipples   Some nipples are dimpled and the end of the nipple, which in most women stands out a tiny bit at least, actually turns inwards. The majority of these inverted nipples can be made to stand out a little more with stimulation, but a few are 'stuck', and are actually kept in place by adhesions under the skin. For some women both nipples are affected; others are only like this on one 'side'. Inverted nipples can make breastfeeding more difficult, and in a very few cases, the struggle is so great that bottle feeding may be the most realistic option (perhaps with expressed breast milk although doing this over a long period may present problems of its own). The baby needs something to latch onto, in order to start the flow of milk (see LATCHING ON; LET-DOWN REFLEX) and inverted nipples may not give him enough. You can help your nipples stand out by wearing BREAST SHELLS in pregnancy and between feeds. Gentle stretching of the nipple – by placing the tip of the index finger on each hand at the edges of the areola and pressing inwards and outwards – may help to break down adhesions. If inverted nipples have stopped you breastfeeding with one baby, it may not mean that you can never breastfeed. Just as flat nipples improve in shape, so inverted nipples may get better during a further pregnancy.

Cracked or sore nipples   I'm dealing with these two topics together, because although soreness doesn't always lead to cracks appearing, cracks almost always start with soreness. Sore/cracked nipples are one of the most common problems associated with breastfeeding. Many women who would otherwise have loved to feed their babies give up in despair because they cannot cope with the pain and the struggle any more. The condition is truly misery-making. Imagine what it's like, having looked forward to this baby throughout pregnancy, to get to the stage where you're dreading the next time she wakes up for a feed and having to offer yourself to her and yet wanting to pull away to avoid the pain.

141

Your nipples are just about the most sensitive areas of skin on your body, and they can become traumatised after only a few feeds, so anything you can do to avoid the problem developing in the first place is far better than curing it once it's there. It should be said that a bit of discomfort in the nipples is normal for many women in the early days of feeding, probably because the nipples might take a few feeds to get used to the new sensation, and the baby needs that time to get used to being 'on' properly. But the soreness should get better, not worse, as time goes on. If it doesn't, something is wrong. Do seek HELP AND ADVICE if you get sore, and at the very least check the position of your baby yourself, because it's now becoming crystal clear that the major cause of sore nipples in breastfeeding is a poor position of the baby on the breast (see LATCHING ON). Get the baby's position right and you won't get sore. And when you want your baby to release your nipple before she drops it herself, break the suction by placing your finger between your nipple and her mouth – never pull her off.

There are other solutions to the problem that are sometimes put forward. Many of them have disadvantages to mother and/or baby. Some of them make the problem worse. Restricting feeds, so that the time on the breast, and therefore the trauma, is lessened is rather pointless. A feed lasting no more than a minute can be painful and damaging to a nipple if the baby isn't fixed on right. In any case, restricting the feeds may lead to less stimulation of the breast, less milk and a hungry, distressed baby. However, always offering the least sore side first is a sort of 'restriction' that may be helpful, as the baby will suck less hard once he's had his first hunger pangs settled by the first breast, and this may make the sucking less painful to the mother.

Applying creams and sprays to the sore or cracked nipple is something many mothers do, and some report that this helps. Yet to be sure your baby isn't going to ingest these substances (and given the choice, you wouldn't really want your baby to eat sheep fat, chemicals, petroleum jelly or whatever you're using), you need to be certain that the substance has had time to sink right into your skin before she's put to the breast again, or else you'll have to rub it or wash it off, which might be painful. I am particularly sceptical of antiseptic sprays, which mothers are supposed to use on the nipple before feeding. Taste and smell one of these on your hand and you'll see how it masks your own scent and taste, and getting used to and fond of these two elements is part of the way your baby learns to feed. Moreover, how sure are we that taking in antiseptics with the breast milk is safe for a baby? Any potion or cream you put on your nipple may cause a reaction in you, because you're sensitive to one or more of the ingredients. This is at least partly why some creams seem to make the problem actually worse. Applying a little expressed breast milk itself to the sore nipple and allowing it to dry is said to promote healing but again, even touching your nipple might be painful. This remedy may be worth trying as at least it can't do any harm. EXPRESSING BREAST MILK a little immediately before a feed may soften the breast enough for the baby to latch on better, too, especially if the nipple is flattish or small. Experiment with different ways of holding your baby (see POSITION AT BREAST) as this will give the sore area a rest, and possibly a chance to heal.

It may be worth totally resting the breast (or breasts – sore nipples usually strike on both sides although not always with the same severity) when the pain is especially bad. This gives you a rest from the pain, and a chance to have some time when you don't dread the next feed. But if you do this, you have to express your milk in order to maintain your supply, and then feed it to your baby by spoon or bottle. If you use a pump to express, stop using it at once if it's painful and use your hand instead as this is much more gentle, and the nipple isn't pulled as it is with a suction pump. Badly cracked nipples can take days to heal; others may only need as little as 12 to 24 hours. When you put your baby back on, pay special attention to the way she's fixed as the fact that your nipples have healed once is no guarantee that they've toughened up enough to withstand poor latching on. You can get sore, and cracked, again. NIPPLE SHIELDS are, in my view, a last resort.

Cracked nipples may or may not bleed and the cracks themselves aren't always visible to the naked eye so even the most tear-jerking soreness may not have anything to show for itself. Some positional errors, though, cause the nipples to develop little blood-coloured stripes where the baby's jaws or tongue have damaged them. Cracks often appear at these points. Persistent or recurrent soreness or cracks may need a medical check.

143

It could be that you have thrush of the nipple, and if you do, both you and your baby need treatment, or you'll continue merrily passing the wretched thing backwards and forwards between you. THRUSH is a common cause of sore nipples in mothers of older babies, who are unlikely to have positioning difficulties. Cracks can develop an underlying infection, and if this persists, it can allow infection to take hold within the breast itself. This may sometimes be an explanation of why some women suffer breast pain, which radiates back from the nipple and which occurs between and during feeds. Other causes of persistent soreness I have come across include eczema on the nipple, and more simply, a reaction to some detergent or fabric conditioner which makes the mother feel itchy or sore. Lastly, TEETHING sometimes causes nipple soreness because a baby's saliva changes, and this has some effect on the skin of the nipple. Rinsing your nipples in plain water after a feed will help.

As with any attempts to heal a sore area, whatever the cause of your sore or cracked nipples, keep them dry and allow air to circulate if you can. This means avoiding soggy BREAST PADS, and when you can, wearing no top clothing. Sunbathe topless if you can, and the sunlight and fresh air will help you too.

NIPPLE SHIELDS

A nipple shield is a covering, usually made of rubber, occasionally plastic and rubber, that's worn over sore or cracked NIPPLES. The idea behind it is that the shield reduces the trauma on the nipple while the baby is feeding, which is supposed to speed up healing. There are disadvantages to using a nipple shield which you should know about before you decide to use one. It has been shown that milk flow is reduced when the mother is wearing a nipple shield, because the shield cuts down on the direct stimulation of the nipple by the baby's mouth. The result of this is that the overall milk supply is reduced. The baby also has to exert greater effort while feeding. This will mean nothing more than longer feeds for a big, healthy baby, but for a smaller, newer one, perhaps one who has a tendency to sleepiness, the effort may mean he falls asleep before he's filled his tummy, and this in turn will reduce the stimulation of the milk supply.

The other major disadvantage is that a nipple shield teaches the baby nothing about breastfeeding. He learns to 'shield-feed', and because new babies learn fast, he gets to prefer to feed with the shield, and loses the technique of feeding from the nipple. In other words, he gets 'hooked' on it. You might end up having to use a shield all the time, simply because your baby won't feed without it. (And at the same time, he mightn't be gaining sufficient weight because he's not able to get enough milk through the shield.) This is fiddly, and negates much of the convenience of breastfeeding as you have to keep the nipple shield sterilised between feeds, take it with you wherever you go, fix it on when you'd prefer to be discreet about breastfeeding, replace it with a clean one if you accidentally drop in on the floor . . . They can harbour organisms like THRUSH; they taste rubbery, or else of the solution they were sterilised in, and therefore condition the baby incorrectly in this way, too (see STERILISATION). They fall off in the middle of a feed, dripping milk everywhere. All in all, there's not a lot of use for them!

If you have sore or cracked nipples there are practical measures which will change the way you are breastfeeding and the position of your baby at the breast, which will help you far more than a nipple shield. In some occasional circumstances, a nipple shield may help an individual woman if the pain of feeding is too much to cope with, and both mum and baby are slow to get the hang of re-positioning (see POSTION AT BREAST). At least the shield gives her a break from the soreness. Don't use it more than a few times; try to remove it when your baby takes a natural break from the breast and before he goes back on, too.

If your baby's already hooked on the shield, and you want to give it up, don't despair too much. It can take a bit of effort and determination to wean him off it, and occasionally babies take the initiative themselves and suddenly get back on the breast without you even thinking about it. Start by offering the shield-less breast at every feed. If your baby insists on the shield, let him start the feed with it, and then try to slip it off when your baby takes a break in feeding. If you don't manage to get him off it, then breastfeeding with a shield is better than not breastfeeding at all despite its problems. So it might be better for you just to give in gracefully and stick with it rather than facing the problem at every feedtime.

NUTS*

Nuts aren't safe for infants and toddlers unless they are ground as the risk of inhaling is too great. They are potential allergens, too, and if you think your baby may suffer from FOOD INTOLERANCE you should avoid nuts in any form until after the first year (see also ALLERGY). Otherwise, ground nuts are a good source of protein and you can give them to your baby from the second stage of WEANING, quite happily.

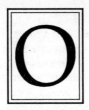

OATS*

Oats contain just a little GLUTEN, and so they are best left until after your baby can cope with first stage foods and they make a good second 'starter' cereal after rice. Most babies like porridge oats, even made with water. Whole oats, known as groats, rather than oat flakes, need more cooking to make them digestible for babies, but they have the advantage of being unmilled, and therefore all the nutrients are retained.

When? From the second stage of WEANING.

OFFAL*

This is the term we use for the animal organs we eat as meat – LIVER, heart, kidneys, tongue and so on. They are especially rich in iron and B vitamins. Offal is suitable for babies who are ready to progress from the first stage of WEANING. Start with lamb's offal and then go on to beef (and ox) and then chicken. You need to make sure the offal you serve isn't too tough, and that any hard-to-digest membranes (for example, in kidneys) have been cut away.

OILS

Oil is liquid fat which is obtained from various sources, including vegetables, nuts and grains. Some are healthier than others – an oil from a single source – for example, sunflower oil, corn oil or soya oil, which are high in polyunsaturates – is preferable to an oil labelled 'vegetable oil'. There is likely to have been less processing involved as the vegetable oil will have come from several different sources and may well contain saturated fat.

Babies find fatty foods hard to digest (see FAT), and you should keep your baby's intake of oil to a minimum. If he has salad, don't dress it in oil. Heating oil to a very high temperature so that it smokes changes its structure, and some experts believe this is harmful to health. So the best advice is to avoid frying your baby's food although stir frying, which needs a lower temperature, should be fine.

ONION

Onions can be introduced as a second-stage vegetable, but they do need to be well-cooked, either by boiling or cooked along with other foods in a casserole. Not all babies like onion though it could be the texture rather than the taste that puts them off. Chopped very finely, onion could well be more acceptable.

When? From the second stage of WEANING.

ORANGE JUICE

See JUICE

ORANGES

Oranges – peeled and pipped – can be given as finger food to babies who can hold the pieces, or chopped up very small to a younger baby. However, only the sweeter varieties are suitable, unless your baby likes sharp tastes. Don't introduce oranges before the second stage of WEANING, or the age of six months, whichever is the later, as they are commonly linked to FOOD INTOLERANCE.

OVERWEIGHT

See WEIGHT

OXYTOCIN

Oxytocin is the hormone responsible for the LET-DOWN REFLEX that allows the breast milk stored in the milk cells to be released down the ducts for the baby. In the days after the birth, you might feel afterpains as your uterus contracts as you feed, due to the presence of oxytocin in your blood stream.

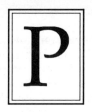

PAEDIATRICIAN

A doctor specialising in the health of babies and children.
See HELP AND ADVICE

PARSNIPS*

Parsnips are a vegetable with a natural sweetness that babies
enjoy. Wash, scrape and chop the parsnips before cooking, and
serve as a mash, a purée or in small pieces as finger food,
according to the age and dexterity of your baby.

When? From the first stage of WEANING.

PARTY FOODS*

Party foods don't have to be junk foods, and at the age of a year,
you really can start good habits, as your baby and his chums,
even those as old as three, won't yet have any expectations.
Serve fruit juice instead of soft drinks or squash. Most toddlers
find ice cubes terribly exciting (though make sure the drinks are
drunk with a straw or through a spouted cup – ice cubes could
cause choking if swallowed whole). Sandwiches should be tiny
and manageable, try fillings such as mashed banana, tuna fish,
egg and tomato and grated cheese. Crisps and savoury 'snacks'
are generally too salty – although some varieties are available
these days which are without salt. Cheese straws are quick to
bake, and babies and children of all ages like them. Sweet foods,
such as little buns and the birthday cake itself, don't need to be
banned. You can try our idea for a birthday cake that isn't full of
the 'wrong' ingredients instead, and use the same mixture for
small cakes, too.

PASTA*

Most pasta is based on wheat, and as long as your baby can tolerate this, he can be given pasta. It's an especially convenient food for babies if you choose it in suitable shapes – butterflies, shells or small macaroni. Long strips of thin spaghetti or tagliatelle are obviously out. Babies can manage to pick up the shapes and eat them as finger foods. Wholemeal pasta is preferable to the 'normal' sort because the whole of the grain is better than the processed, 'white' grain. The taste is better, too.

You can serve pasta with all sorts of meat, vegetables and other foods. Try it with grated cheese on top, plus a vegetable. Remember not to salt the cooking water.

When? From the second stage of WEANING when your baby is already used to wheat in other forms such as bread. *Or* it can be used as an introduction to wheat-based foods.

PASTRY

Pastry is usually made with wheat flour, though you can make it with other flours instead. It's more nutritious made with wholegrain flour but if the results you get are too stodgy for your taste, you can compromise and use half white, half wholegrain flours. You normally need a pinch of salt in a pastry mixture to bring out the flavour and a tiny amount like this isn't going to harm your baby, so don't worry. Pastry off-cuts, can be baked along side the main dish and your baby can have them as finger food. Form the off-cuts into different shapes – circles, little people, long worms – for added interest.

When? From the second stage of WEANING, or when your baby can cope with wheat.

PATÉ

Paté is not suitable for babies and young toddlers because of the high proportion of FAT, SALT and preservatives in it (see also ADDITIVES AND COLOURINGS).

151

PEACHES & NECTARINES*

Peel peaches and nectarines before giving them to your baby. You can mash the flesh, or else give it to him in slivers or cubes as finger food, and it's nice mixed in with yoghurt. Canned peaches seem to be a basic element in the British diet, but they aren't suitable for babies because the sugar content of the syrup is very high. You can get cans of peaches in a sugar-free liquid, but they still won't be as good as the real thing.

When? From the second stage of WEANING.

PEANUT BUTTER

Use peanut butter sparingly for babies under a year. It's a good source of concentrated protein, but it's also very high in fat. Avoid the varieties with sugar and salt in them (more likely to be available in wholefood or health shops).

When? From the second stage of WEANING.

PEANUTS

See NUTS

PEAS*

Fresh or frozen peas are best for your baby. Canned varieties usually have salt, sugar or green colourings in them. Peas make good finger food, and babies coming up to a year old can usually manage to cope with picking them up between finger and thumb, or mashed, when they can be spooned. A quick idea for lunch is to add a few peas to the cooking water when you are preparing pasta or rice for your baby (the length of time you need to allow depends on whether they're fresh or frozen – fresh peas take about 10 minutes; frozen, about four). Serve the pasta/rice and peas with grated cheese on top.

When? From the second stage of WEANING.

PEPPERS

Cook peppers by boiling, steaming or with other foods in a casserole. Rather like onion, peppers aren't especially liked by babies, at least in my experience. They do need to be chopped finely, because the skin can be a bit tough for babies who aren't good at chewing.

When? From the second stage of WEANING.

PERIODS

See MENSTRUATION

PINEAPPLE

Like peaches, tinned pineapple's a British favourite, but only the varieties canned without a sugary syrup are suitable for babies. Fresh pineapple is better anyway, and easy to prepare. Pineapple flesh needs no cooking, but it's probably too tough for most babies under a year to cope with unless it's mashed well or puréed. Mix the mashed flesh with yoghurt, or serve it with a spoon of yoghurt on top.

When? From the second stage of WEANING.

PKU

Phenylketonuria is the full name for this rare metabolic disorder and it is generally known as PKU. About one baby in 10,000 is affected, and babies in the UK are given a routine blood test known as the Guthrie test or the heel-prick test to detect it. It's an inherited inability to produce a vital enzyme needed in digestion. Once detected, brain damage is only avoided by adherence to a special diet.

PLATES

Plastic plates are best for your baby as they are virtually unbreakable – although I have a soft spot for china 'bunny plates', despite their lack of practicality! Choose plates with raised sides, bowl-shaped or like an old-fashioned 'porringer', which makes spooning the food that much easier, and the food less likely to fall off the edge during the meal. Some plates can be bought with a suction pad that you stick to the high chair tray, this prevents the plate from being thrown or otherwise pushed off the edge of the tray. I've heard too many stories and witnessed too many babies pushing up against the suction so that it finally breaks, tipping the food onto the floor with great force, so I don't feel I could recommend them. They may suit a baby who hasn't cottoned on to the suction principle yet, of course.

A stay-warm plate can be used with an enclosed reservoir of hot water underneath the food section. This is designed to keep the food warm throughout the meal. In my experience, babies don't care about the temperature of their food as long as it's not too hot for them, so I fail to see the benefit of this device. Nevertheless, maybe your baby's extra fussy about cold food!

PLUMS & PRUNES*

Plums should be cooked for babies under a year, unless they're very small, tender and sweet. Peel them, stone them and chop, stewing in a small pan with very little water. You may need to sweeten the result to make it palatable – apple juice is a better alternative to sugar.

Stewed prunes have connotations of school dinners for adults, but your baby is totally unprejudiced about them and may actually like them. Buy ready-to-eat dried prunes and cook them in water until they're plump and tender. Chop and serve, or purée if necessary. Prune juice is a tried and tested remedy for constipation, and worth trying before getting laxatives from the doctor.

When? From the second stage of WEANING.

PORRIDGE*

Porridge is a cooked mix of CEREALS and milk or water. We usually think of porridge as being made from oats, but it doesn't have to be. You can try it with oatmeal, rice, rye, or barley, for example. The rice given to babies as a starter solid is a porridge of sorts. It's actually very easy to make your own porridge from different grains. Adults and older children can share in it, too, which makes it a convenient family breakfast. Flaked grains take less time to cook than the unflaked grains. Don't give porridge with sugar mixed in. If you feel your baby doesn't like it without some sort of sweetening or flavouring, then you could add fresh or dried fruit, puréeing the mixture if you need to.

When? Rice and other grains which are free from GLUTEN (for example, millet) can be used at the first stage of WEANING. Then move on to oats, and then wheat.

POSITION AT BREAST

Don't feel worried if you're 'all thumbs' when you first try BREASTFEEDING. It can be difficult to get a position that feels comfortable, natural and effective, even if you've breastfed before. Resolve to yourself that you'll get some help in positioning and LATCHING ON, and accept that it may take several feeds, and days, before you feel you've got it absolutely right each time.

You don't have to feed in the same position each time. The important thing is that your baby's face and body should be close to your breast and in the same line. She shouldn't have to feed 'over her shoulder', which would be the case, for example, if she lay on her back in your arms, turning her head to face the breast. That's something that older babies sometimes do because they may get to the stage where they can feed in just about any position, but for a new baby it's a recipe for sore NIPPLES at the very least, and a failing milk supply at worst. Your baby's head needs to be tilted very slightly back. If she points her chin towards her chest, she won't be able to latch on well. Her chin should touch your breast, and her mouth should be centred on your nipple. Support her well, down the length of her body. This will keep her well-positioned and close to you without effort, so don't just hold her head and her feet, leaving the rest of her body to slump down. Again, older babies might manage well if you do this; younger babies will tend to drag on the nipple. You can give this support with your arms, or if you're lying down, your baby can rest on one arm, or be supported by the bed itself, or the

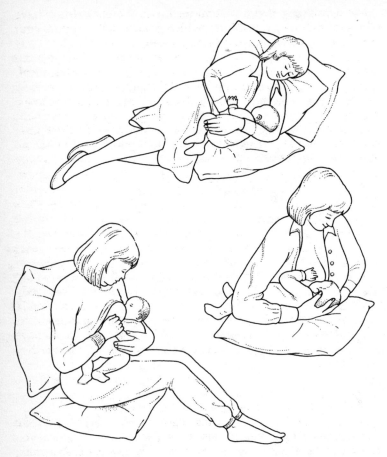

Positions for breastfeeding

Make sure that you are both comfortable. You may like to read, watch television or listen to music. Lying down can be relaxing, especially if you have had a Caesarean section and if you want to feed your baby in bed at night. If you sit up when you are breastfeeding, see that your back is supported and hold the baby high enough so that you don't have to hunch. If you have twins or sore nipples you could try the 'twins hold', sometimes known as the 'rugby ball hold' with a baby under each arm. As long as babies are well supported (with pillows and cushions if necessary) and their faces and bodies are close to you, this position is as good as any other.

crook of your arm if you're semi-reclining. It often helps to have plenty of pillows or cushions, which in turn will support your arms and prevent you from getting tired.

In hospital, sitting on the edge of a bed feeding – as we so often do – is not a helpful start. Nor are the usual hospital chairs ideal, as they are straight backed and relatively high-legged. You really need to either sit or lie back in bed, supported by lots of pillows, and with a pillow under your arms, or, if you do sit in the chair, you need at least one pillow across your lap. Once you're home, you'll have a better choice of seating. Maybe a relative has an old-fashioned nursing chair to lend which has a seat that's only inches off the floor, so that your thighs become a good, support-ive lap when you're sitting on it. The 'conventional' position of baby across your body, legs pointing away from the breast she's on, is the one that most women adopt most of the time in the end, though they may always lie down for NIGHT FEEDS. It's comfortable for both you and the baby, and it has the advantage that you can feed relatively discreetly in public, which is impor-tant to some of us. This is because, with clothing raised to expose the breast, the baby hides the nipple, and the rest of her body hides any exposed midriff. After a couple of weeks, you're unlikely to need cushions and pillows, or even much thought, as you and your baby find out what suits you both best. If you have sore nipples, trying out different positions may help while they are healing.

POTATO*

Mashed potato is a good starter vegetable for a baby when she comes to mixed feeding. It's also versatile because, like rice, you can mix it with other foods. You can mix it with breast milk, formula milk, with other vegetables when it comes to expanding her repertoire, with cheese, egg, gravy . . . and so on. Chunks of cold boiled potato make good finger food. Babies seem to like the taste of potato, and this liking stays with them later – very few toddlers and children get fussy about it. You can boil the potatoes in their skins and then peel before mashing them (the skin tends to fall off), and if a bit of peel remains, it won't matter. As your baby gets older, she'll be able to cope more easily with peel and as potatoes are more nutritious this way she'll be getting more vitamins. New potatoes don't ever need more than a wash and a slight scrape.

What about chips, roast or fried potatoes? Babies old enough to chew on them (say from nine months on) won't be harmed by them if they are given occasionally, and chopped if necessary. You need to make sure they're not especially greasy.

When? Mashed or puréed potatoes from the first stage of WEANING. Fried/roast potatoes: occasionally from nine months.

POWDERED MILK

The only sort of powdered (dried) milk suitable for babies is a specially-modified FORMULA MILK. Other dried milks are skimmed milks, lacking in vitamins and fat, which are an essential part of milk for all babies and young children.

PREMATURE BABY

See PRE-TERM BABY

PRESSURE COOKER

See EQUIPMENT

PRE-TERM BABY

A baby born before 37 weeks of pregnancy is pre-term. The other description is premature, but pre-term is gradually taking over. A pre-term baby has very special feeding needs. He may not be able to suck and swallow in a properly co-ordinated way, for example, and he may need to be fed by tube. Exactly what he should be fed on is still the subject of research. Because pre-term babies so easily lose weight, and yet need to grow in order to increase their strength, it's been thought by some that formula milk feeding, with a formula constituted for pre-term infants, is the best course. Pre-term babies do generally gain weight faster on formula, it's true. However, pre-term babies are at a greater risk of infection, and benefit greatly from the protective factors in breast milk. There is more to feeding pre-term babies than 'fill him up and watch him grow'.

Mothers of pre-term infants produce milk that's more concentrated than the milk of full-term infants, though it is usually in tiny quantities at first. Because the baby may not be able to suck from the breast, the milk is expressed and then given by tube. Tiny babies can't take a lot of food at once anyway, so the small amounts produced by the mother may be enough. In other cases the stress of the situation, the difficulty experienced by mothers in EXPRESSING BREAST MILK (which is often not as effective a way of building up a milk supply as a feeding baby), and poor information from hospital staff, who may not think that breast-feeding's a realistic option, lead to insufficient milk, and the shortfall has to be made up with formula milk (later the breast MILK SUPPLY can be increased, especially once the baby is able to suck).

Many pre-term babies go from tube feeding to bottle feeding and then on to attempted breastfeeding (see CHANGING: FROM BOTTLE TO BREAST). It's done this way because breast-feeding is supposed to be more difficult for the baby and he's likely to tire himself out until he's bigger and stronger. In fact, breastfeeding is likely to be *easier* for the baby. Once the LET-DOWN REFLEX works, all the baby has to do is to swallow, keeping up the flow with only occasional sucks. The milk comes down by itself, with minimum effort on the baby's part. Of course, the breastfeeding mother of a pre-term baby needs a lot of support and encouragement. We know that her feelings after giving birth so soon and unexpectedly can be confused and even guilty. She might not trust her body and it can be frightening to feel totally responsible for a tiny little scrap who looks as though he might break if held too close. Staff need to boost her confidence in breastfeeding, explain why it's worth doing, and to help her get herself comfortable, and the baby well-positioned at the breast, every time.

Expressing milk regularly and often, at least six times a day or more if possible, with an electric pump or by hand (whichever's the most productive) needs motivation. Meanwhile, the baby can come to the breast even before he's able to feed directly as he needs to learn about the smell, security and warmth he can have from his mother. This will help him breastfeed later. In some

159

units, babies are given the milk they need in addition to breast milk by means of spouted cups, that pour the milk into the mouth in small quantities. This means the baby never gets to learn about 'bottle sucking' and never runs the risk of nipple confusion. This can happen when a baby is unable to feed from the breast because his sucking technique only works with a rubber teat. Human milk from a milk bank can be used to supplement the mother's own milk. Research done on human milk enriched with extra minerals to make a sort of 'human formula milk' looks promising, and babies fed on this, plus their mother's milk, grow just as well as those on cow's milk formula.

If you want to breastfeed your pre-term baby, then be assured that it's possible, and that it's important. Hold him close to you whenever you can take him out of his perspex box, and seek the help and co-operation of the hospital staff, too. Breastfeeding counsellors will also help (see HELP AND ADVICE). If it doesn't work out, and you find it's becoming too much of a struggle, you may want to switch to the bottle instead (see CHANGING: FROM BREAST TO BOTTLE).

PROLACTIN

When your baby sucks at the breast, nerve endings respond by 'telling' the pituitary gland to produce the hormone prolactin. Prolactin is the 'milk-making' hormone, and it's under its influence that the milk cells continue to make milk to feed your baby. Interestingly, prolactin levels are highest during sleep, which is at least part of the reason why many women feel very 'full' in the mornings. Prolactin levels in mothers using a pump to express their milk are apparently low, compared with mothers feeding their babies directly. This partly explains why it can be very difficult to establish and maintain a MILK SUPPLY when the only stimulation comes from EXPRESSING BREAST MILK. Prolactin suppresses ovulation, which is why breastfeeding has a contraceptive effect. See CONTRACEPTION

PROTEIN

Protein is made up of different amino acids, some of which are known as 'essential amino acids' as they cannot be made by the body, but need to be present in the diet. Foods containing protein are needed for growth, and to maintain the health of the body tissue and the blood. The body can't store protein very efficiently, so we need a daily intake. The protein present in breast milk is just right for an infant; some brands of formula milk have had their protein content modified to make them more suitable for a baby's digestion. When a baby moves on to mixed feeding, his protein needs will still be served by milk, in the main, but he will also be getting supplies in cereals, cheese, eggs, meat, fish, beans and pulses. Vegetables and fruits contain some protein, too. We tend to put a great emphasis on protein, worrying in case our children are not getting enough. In fact, it's very difficult for a baby or toddler to go short of protein if he drinks milk, as this and many of our most common foods including the ones we give to babies, contain protein. You need to take care if you are weaning your baby onto a vegan diet, in order to maintain sufficient protein in your baby's diet from plant sources (see VEGANISM).

PRUNES

See PLUMS AND PRUNES

PUDDINGS

See DESSERTS

PULSES

See BEANS AND PULSES

PURÉES

This describes a way of cooking and straining (or blending or food processing) that reduces the food to a manageable sort of pulp, which is then spoon-fed to a baby. It can be a mistake to only ever offer purées to your baby as she can get too used to perfect smoothness and become very conservative about accepting anything else. This is one of the major disadvantages of BABY FOODS, in my view. Even if you're starting your baby off on solids at the lower end of the acceptable age range, say between four and four and a half months, it's likely that she'll manage a bit of lumpiness, as long as she can suck it in without being expected to chew with toothless gums!

PYLORIC STENOSIS

This is a condition occurring in about one in every 500 babies. It's caused by a thickening of the tissues at the place where the stomach meets the intestine, this narrows the outlet and the stomach's contents can't easily pass through. The result is that the baby vomits after every feed, and the VOMITING gets worse over a period, until it becomes 'projectile', shooting out several feet. This is different from the sort of vomiting seen in a 'SICKY' BABY, who may be sick because his stomach is too full, but nothing like as forcefully. A baby with pyloric stenosis will fail to thrive and needs to be seen by a doctor. A simple operation to open the outlet cures the condition permanently.

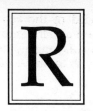

R

RAISINS AND SULTANAS

For a young baby, you can soak raisins or sultanas for a few hours and then stew until the fruit is tender (about ten minutes) and it is worth keeping the liquid as a sweetener for dishes such as porridge. Dried, uncooked raisins and sultanas are not suitable for babies under a year as they could easily be swallowed whole, causing CHOKING. They are also sticky and sugary, so look upon them as you would ordinary SWEETS. Always rinse raisins and sultanas well before using them, because most brands are coated in a potentially harmful mineral oil to keep them moist.

RASPBERRIES

See BERRIES

REHEATING FOOD

See LEFT-OVERS

RELACTATION

All women who have ever had a baby can, in theory, start up their milk supply once more. You need motivation, support and usually a co-operative baby! The longer it is since you last breastfed, the more difficult it's likely to be, but if you want to do it, then have a go. Occasionally, mothers who adopt a child years after breastfeeding their own manage to begin feeding again, and there are a few documented cases of adoptive mothers who have never even been pregnant managing to produce milk, in quite large quantities, too.
See also CHANGING: FROM BOTTLE TO BREAST

RHUBARB

Cooked rhubarb is usually too tart to be given to a baby without being sweetened. Try adding concentrated apple juice rather than sugar. Alternatively, serve it with another, more naturally sweet fruit such as a sweet apple, perhaps grated finely. You do need to cook rhubarb well, and chop or mash it finely, to make it easy for a baby to digest.

When? Rhubarb contains oxalic acid, so leave it until your baby is six months old.

RICE*

Rice is a grain that is free of GLUTEN, it is easy to digest and low on any list of potential causes of FOOD INTOLERANCE. This is why it's often a baby's first cereal, and in fact, often the baby's first introduction to any food other than milk. You don't have to give rice at the start of weaning – fruits and vegetables might be easier for you, instead. Some rice is commercially-packaged and marketed as 'baby rice', or under some well known proprietary name such as Farlene or Farex. Rice is brown or white, ground or flaked, or in the form of flour. All the widely-available baby rices are white, and they may have vitamins added to them as well. Choose one without added milk powder or sugar. Brown rice is more nutritious than white because it contains the whole of the grain. This isn't a crucial difference at first; a baby takes such a very small amount of rice that his major source of nutrition is still his milk, whether it is breast or formula, and the 'missing' vitamins in white rice aren't important. The difference in FIBRE content is not important, either, at this stage.

The major advantage of baby rice is that it's prepared instantly – mix it with liquid and there you are. If you want to use ordinary brown rice, and find the preparation-time off-putting, buy ground brown rice or rice flour – it takes no more than a few minutes to prepare. Rice that you've prepared for the family can be puréed (adding more liquid if necessary) and served to your baby (remember not to salt the rice while cooking – leave the salt until after you've removed the baby's portion). You can mix the rice you give your baby with expressed breast milk, formula milk or water (or later, ordinary full-fat pasteurised milk), whatever sort it is. Because rice mixes so easily with many other foods, it's a good thickener for purées and mashes. You can serve it with vegetables, fruit or meat, and it can be a help in making unfamiliar food familiar to a baby who seems to have conservative tastes.

Rice cakes (they can be bought sugar and salt free) are available in health and wholefood shops and are a good alternative to ordinary rusks. Most babies like them a lot, and they seem to make less mess than rusks!

When? From the first stage of WEANING.

ROOTING REFLEX

A baby is born with a strong instinct to feed from his mother's breast, and this can be seen in the rooting reflex. If you stroke a new baby's cheek, the reflex causes him to turn his head in the direction of the stroking finger and start to open his mouth.

ROUTINES

If you like a routine in your daily life, if you've heard that babies need one, that they get distressed if they're 'out of their routine', or if you can't imagine life with a baby without some sort of predictability in it, then you might be dismayed when you hear about the importance of 'feeding on demand', or 'letting the baby set the pace'. Let me reassure you. If routine is important to you and, let's face it, few of us have lives we can devote entirely to our babies' needs, then you'll be able to achieve it. Just don't expect it to happen in the first week or so, that's all! But, feeding your baby when he wants is important in getting your MILK SUPPLY established (see DEMAND FEEDING). But this regime needn't go on forever. For a start, babies often develop a predictability of their own as they space their feeds out. If this doesn't happen after a few weeks you can impose a little order on the chaos by doing one or more of several things:
• always waking the baby in the morning and feeding at the hour which suits you and your family (you'll have to keep it up at weekends if you want it to really stick!), even on the occasions

when he wakes at six and then goes back to sleep. If it suits you to wake him at seven, and start the day then, go ahead.

• having a bedtime routine that takes place at approximately the same time every night, for example, a feed, followed by playtime (babies are often wakeful in the early evening), bathtime, followed by a further, longer feed.

• having separate sleeping places for day-time and night-time (perhaps the carrycot downstairs in the day, and the crib upstairs at night). This sometimes helps babies who have their days and nights mixed up and wake frequently in the night, and sleep peacefully during the day for long periods. These babies need to be woken up often in the day to feed.

• check that you're allowing your baby to feed as long as he wants from the first side, in order to make sure he gets the more filling HIND MILK as well as the FORE MILK. Changing sides for the sake of it may make him feed more frequently than otherwise, as he gets hungrier, quicker. Although, sometimes frequent 'side-switching' can increase MILK SUPPLY.

• check your baby's always well-positioned on the breast (see LATCHING ON; POSITION AT BREAST).

• if you're happy with your milk supply and your baby's gaining weight and is otherwise healthy, try a dummy, to see if this can satisfy his need to suck without always needing to feed (see DUMMIES, SOOTHERS OR PACIFIERS).

• if he is constantly fussy and unsettled (see COLIC; CRYING; DIET AND BREASTFEEDING).

• bottle fed babies usually get into a routine quicker than breastfeds, because of the fixed amount of milk offered at each feed, and the longer time it takes formula to be digested. If you're bottle feeding and not getting into a routine, use the appropriate suggestions above. Some bottle fed babies need a different formula in order to satisfy them more. Your health visitor will help you decide what's right for you (see HELP AND ADVICE).

• when you think about starting solids, aim to introduce them – even the first tiny tastes – at a time that fits in with what your baby's mealtimes will be (see WEANING).

Remember if your baby's healthy and happy, and you are too, then there's nothing magic about having a routine if you don't want or need one! In any case, any routine should be flexible. There will be days when your baby is hungrier more often. He may be needing more milk to grow at that particular time, maybe he needs the extra fuel to fight an infection that you're not aware of or perhaps he needs comfort and security for some reason. Almost all babies are in a routine when they're having three meals a day, anyway, although they may have extra milk feeds at other times.

RUSKS*

Most commercial rusks are really only biscuits for babies. They mash up well in milk or water, probably better than most ordinary biscuits, and they come in pretty boxes. They may have the odd extra added vitamin or two. But that's it. They are available in varieties which are low in SUGAR, but you do need to treat this with some scepticism. They may be low in sucrose (ordinary white 'table sugar') but have other sugars in them, such as dextrose, glucose or maltose. They will also be made from white flour. Try eating a rusk yourself, low-sugar or otherwise, and you'll taste just how sweet it is. So unless you can find sugar-free rusks, made from wholegrain flour, your baby will be better off having a bought rusk no more often than occasionally. The alternative is to make your own – and it's really very easy – from bread. Rice cakes (see RICE) are available from wholefood and health shops, and make an excellent substitute without being any more expensive.

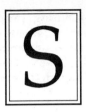

SALADS*

Raw vegetables (sometimes with fruit), chopped and mixed with some sort of dressing (oil, yoghurt or fruit juice, for example) as a salad can be given to your baby in small quantities – though make sure he is able to tolerate the ingredients cooked, first. Raw fruit and vegetables give the digestive system something to work on and that's one of the reasons why they're a healthy complement to cooked foods for older children and adults. But your baby's digestion can gradually work up to that, as he gets used to foods other than milk. Giving a baby under a year raw food is not always advisable, and some raw foods may pass right through the digestive system more or less untouched, which means the baby can't have got much from them.

There are some foods your baby can be introduced to in their raw state, however, in or out of a salad (though remember new foods should be introduced one at a time). These include apple, pear, banana as well as those fruits and vegetables you'd be unlikely to cook such as peaches, lettuce (shred finely) and cucumber (peel). Make sure the salad ingredients you give to your baby are grated or chopped very small, or else in pieces big enough for him to hold and therefore too big to be popped in whole. A very light dressing of oil and lemon juice on your baby's salad should be fine although he may actually prefer it without. Alternatively, use a spoon or two of natural yoghurt.

When? After the second stage of WEANING is well-established.

SALT

Salt (sodium chloride) is necessary to life, but an excess of it can be harmful. For a baby, the right amount of salt is obtained in breast milk, and the sodium levels in cow's milk have to be reduced in the manufacturing process of formula milk. A baby's kidneys cannot cope with a high level of salt, and if they're severely overloaded, the result can be severe dehydration, or at worst, kidney damage. The ability to excrete sodium efficiently from the body doesn't develop until toddlerhood, so throughout the first year, your baby should avoid added salt. During weaning, he will get all the salt he needs from his breast or formula milk, and from the amounts naturally present in other foods. This means if you're giving your baby some of the family meal, you'll need to cook it without salt and extract your baby's portion before adding it. Foods such as pre-packed meats, crisps, tinned vegetables, ready-to-eat frozen meals, packet and canned soups and so on generally contain a lot of salt (sometimes in the form of monosodium glutamate), as it acts as a preservative as well as a flavouriser. These foods aren't suitable for your baby.

See ADDITIVES AND COLOURINGS; CONVENIENCE FOODS

SANDWICHES*

Once your baby's old enough to manage finger food, try him with sandwiches occasionally. Cut them up small, if necessary, and you'll find they're convenient, quick to make and, with the right sort of filling, very nutritious.

SCHEDULED FEEDING

Scheduled feeding and breastfeeding don't go together, at least not in the first few weeks while your breast milk supply is becoming established. Some hospitals still recommend to mothers that they feed according to a schedule, usually every four hours. Sometimes, there's some totally arbitrary cut-off line: babies under seven pounds are fed three hourly; those over seven pounds are fed four hourly. This can work with bottle feeding, and in a very few cases a breastfeeding mother may produce enough milk in spite of it, but in the majority of cases, breastfeeding according to a schedule leads to bottle feeding. It's as simple as that. The breasts need stimulating as often as the baby wants to feed, in order to make as much milk

169

as he wants. If this doesn't happen, the milk supply will trail off.

Of course, some babies do adopt a schedule of their own, right from the first few days. That's okay, but if the schedule means you're feeding six times a day or less, then you still may not be giving your breast milk production a chance to get underway. If there's any indication your baby may be gaining weight too slowly, then wake him to feed more often. In fact, the only place for scheduled feeds at the start of breastfeeding is when your baby is sleepy or lacking in the energy to feed; then you may have to clock-watch, to make sure he has at least eight feeds in 24 hours. Later on, a feeding schedule might suit you, and when you're confident your milk supply is established, and your baby is happily gaining weight, you can aim to adopt one, although it's best to remain flexible and be prepared to return to more frequent feeding if needed.

See DEMAND FEEDING; ROUTINES

SEASONING

You should avoid added SALT in your baby's food, but a small amount of herbs and mild spices (that is, not spices such as curry, chili, pepper and mustard) whether dried or fresh, can be used once your baby is eating a variety of foods.

When? From about nine months.

SEEDS*

Seeds, like nuts, are a good source of protein. Babies under a year can be given seeds but they do need to be ground. They can then be sprinkled on porridge, in soups or stews to add extra protein and minerals. You can toast seeds under the grill first and then grind. Try varieties like sunflower seeds, pumpkin seeds and pine kernels.

When? When the second stage of WEANING is established.

SEMI-SKIMMED MILK

See COW'S MILK

SEX AND BREASTFEEDING

You can't actually predict what effect, if any, breastfeeding will have on your sex life, but you can prepare yourself with some information in advance. Because both breastfeeding and sexual excitement initiate a hormonal response when OXYTOCIN is released into the bloodstream, the growing excitement leading up to orgasm and the orgasm itself can mean you leak breast milk. Whether this is a turn-on or a turn-off for you or your partner is up to you! Leaking is less likely if you feed the baby before you make love, which is what you'll probably do at first anyway, as being the only way you can hope for an uninterrupted time together. Wearing a BRA in bed is another possible way to lessen the effects of leaking (see LEAKING FROM BREASTS).

Some women don't feel very 'breast-orientated' during love-making even if they used to be before the baby. If this applies to you, then tell your partner that what you used to like in the way of caresses, sucking and so on is out for the moment and reassure him that your feelings will return (and they will). On the other hand, the increased sensitivity of the breasts at this time may make you feel very positive sensations – tell your partner if that's the case instead! The connection between breastfeeding and sex might be threatening or off-putting to some people. For some men, the idea that their partner is using her breasts in this way makes them feel jealous or embarrassed. It's true to say, too, that if women are embarrassed about their bodies and their femininity, the idea of breastfeeding is going to be a pretty negative one. If you recognise feelings like this in yourself or your partner, and yet there is something within you that wants to breastfeed, then it's worth trying. Your feelings might change when you get going!

The tiredness involved with caring for a new baby may lessen your sex drive, and this may be nothing to do with whether you breastfeed or not. It could be that because breastfeeding is such a close, warm experience, a woman's need for intimacy is at least partly satisfied by the experience, and so sex becomes less important. Others feel more ready for sex, perhaps because breastfeeding enhances their body-awareness and subtly stimulates them sexually, too. If you find breastfeeding is a mildly or even strongly sexual experience (and there are reports of women having orgasms during a feed . . .), don't feel in anyway abnormal. And don't feel abnormal if you find it nothing more than a pleasant and relaxing way to feed your baby, either. If your partner likes the idea of getting milk from your breasts himself, then he can if you don't mind either.

Breastfeeding has a contraceptive effect, but if you want to avoid conception for sure, you'll need to avoid intercourse or else use some kind of CONTRACEPTION.

See also FATHERS AND BREASTFEEDING

SHARON FRUIT

The pulp of the sharon fruit can be mashed or sieved and given to a baby on a spoon. You can also mix it with other foods such as cottage cheese or yoghurt.

When? From the second stage of WEANING.

SICKNESS

See ILLNESS; VOMITING

'SICKY' BABY

A 'sicky' baby is not the same as a 'sickly' baby, which implies the baby is ailing in some way. A 'sicky' baby is one who is healthy and happy and who feeds well, but who often brings up a lot of her milk. She will bring up large amounts after every feed, and between feeds she's likely to be dribbling and drooling half-digested milk. It doesn't seem to bother her, and if it goes on for more than a few weeks, it may even appear as if she likes doing it. It can happen to breast fed babies, but it's more common in bottle fed babies. It's a big nuisance, as the constant mopping up and clothes-changing can get you down. If this happens to your baby, have her checked over medically to rule out any underlying problem. Then get on with coping with the practical side. Swathe yourself and your baby in nappies or towels; avoid juggling or moving her abruptly during her feed or immediately afterwards. See if keeping her upright for ten or 15 minutes after she's finished will help. If your baby wears a bib more or less all the time it will save you having to change clothing quite so often. The moving about when you undress and dress her could make the problem worse, anyway. Babies like this do usually improve after three months or so, and the problem rarely remains as bad as the baby gets to be able to sit up by herself.

SKIMMED MILK

See COW'S MILK

SLEEPING

See COLIC; CRYING; NIGHT FEEDS

SLEEPY BABY

Many new babies are sleepy – and thank goodness for that, say many parents. However, some babies are jaundiced, tired after a long and difficult birth, affected by pain killers the mum took in labour, small . . . and any of these factors can make the baby too sleepy for her own good. She may need to be woken for feeds if you wish to establish a good milk supply, and also to help her grow. If after the first week or so, you're not breastfeeding at least six to eight times a day and you are having difficulty keeping your baby awake during the feeds, or if you're feeding on demand and your baby is not gaining WEIGHT well enough because she sleeps, apparently contentedly, for long periods, you should aim to wake her up more often. Keep her awake by changing her nappy in the middle of the feed, stroking her tummy, switching her from one side to the other and back again, and by unwrapping any warm clothing she may have on. Don't let her have a dummy which can soothe her to sleep again every time she stirs to wake. Any of these suggestions can be used with a bottle fed baby who needs to feed more.

SMOKING

A smoky atmosphere is an unhealthy one for a young baby, so if you or your partner smoke, and can't give it up, then try to smoke in a room where the baby doesn't normally sleep, eat or feed. This isn't always practical, though, and it could be that giving up is easier in the long term. Nicotine does get through to the breast milk, and smoking can also reduce the quantity of milk you produce, which are further disadvantages to a new baby. Of course, you will need help and support to give up smoking (I know – I used to smoke and had a hard time, and many failed attempts, at stopping). But the benefits to you and your children will be great.

See COLIC

SNACKS*

When your baby's on solid food, it's unlikely he'll be able to stick to three meals a day, plus drinks, without wanting something in between, at least occasionally. Here are some ideas for healthy snacks:

fruit slice
rice cake
home-made rusk
breadstick
crispbread
cooked carrot finger
cooked potato slice
small piece of cheese
slice/crust of bread
orange segments

SOCIETY AND BREASTFEEDING

Breastfeeding shouldn't ever be seen as something a bit odd – after all, the majority of the world's children are fed in this way, and even in the UK, which has some of the lowest breastfeeding rates in the West, most mothers start off breastfeeding their babies. However, if you do feel odd, or other people who perhaps haven't tried to breastfeed make you feel odd, look for support from other mothers. Join a group or ask your health visitor if she knows of any breastfeeding mums nearby you could chum up with. Read up on the benefits of breastfeeding so you feel bolstered by the fact that you're doing something very positive for your baby (see BOOKLIST).

When you're out visiting, you can breastfeed fairly discreetly with a little practice. Tops that pull up are easier to cope with than dresses or blouses you open down the front. When you're shopping, look out for the Mother & Baby symbol that shows you where there are feeding and changing facilities. Big stores catering for mothers and children are increasingly likely to have specially-equipped rooms for you. Wherever you are, if you don't feel embarrassed about feeding 'in public', then there's no reason why other people's hang-ups should prevent you, unless the fact that they're uncomfortable makes you feel uneasy, too.

Mothers often feel under pressure from close relatives who suggest that the baby 'can't be getting enough', or who can't believe it's possible to totally breastfeed. Feeding babies *is* an emotional area, let's face it. If your mother-in-law is always at you to give bottles, it could be that she's unhappy about the sort of feeding experiences she had ... even 20 or 30 years on. It's highly unlikely that anyone who's had a good breastfeeding experience will be negative about you breastfeeding your baby – so find someone like that and get to know her! It's important to get support from your partner – especially in the early weeks when baby care and feeding can be at its most demanding. Dads can really help with breastfeeding, just by *being* there and sharing in the mother's feelings about it.
See FATHERS AND BREASTFEEDING; HELP AND ADVICE; USEFUL ADDRESSES

SODIUM

See SALT

SOLIDS

Along with most other people, mothers, health visitors, doctors and authors included, I take the word solids to mean any food other than milk – even though it may be anything but actually solid.
See WEANING

SORE NIPPLES

See NIPPLES

SOUP*

It's easy to make your own soup, and it's a meal all members of the family can enjoy, as long as the baby's portion is unsalted. A blender or food processor can make soup out of a selection of already-cooked vegetables; add water if necessary and re-heat. Canned soup is not usually suitable for a baby under a year because of the salt content. Some varieties also have additives and colourings in them, as well as sugar. Packet soup should be avoided for the same reasons. Both canned and packet soups are lower in nutritional value than most home-made soups, too.

When? From the first or second stage of WEANING, depending on the ingredients used.

SOYA MILK

Soya milk is obtained by processing the soya bean. It's free of animal protein and also of lactose (milk sugar), and for this reason it's sometimes given to babies who are intolerant of cow's milk (see FOOD INTOLERANCE). If a baby under six months is to be fed on soya milk, it must be one of the specially-modified formulas. In fact, soya formula should only be used when there's definite reason to suspect cow's milk intolerance. There's no sound reason to think that soya milk is any less likely to cause food intolerance than cow's milk, either. You are still introducing a foreign protein into your baby's diet, albeit a vegetable protein, and this can have the effect of sensitising the baby's gut in the same way as cow's milk protein. If your baby is on formula milk, and has been properly diagnosed (by a paediatrician with a knowledge of allergy) as cow's milk intolerant, then by all means consider using a soya milk formula (though don't reject the possibility of RELACTATION, either). Otherwise, there is no advantage in using it.

SPICES

See SEASONING

SPINACH

The evidence is that spinach is not suitable for babies under six months. It contains a substance called oxalic acid, which affects the absorption of calcium into the body. Other experts recommend its delay because of the way it deteriorates so rapidly after picking. Small quantities of very fresh, perhaps even home-grown, spinach are unlikely to be harmful, however, as the effect on calcium absorption would only be significant with frequent consumption.

SPOONS AND SPOONFEEDING

Chunky, plastic spoons are easiest for a young baby to manage although don't expect anything approaching efficient self-spooning until after the first birthday. You can give your baby the idea by always placing a spoon in her dish, even when you are using another spoon to feed her with. But, of course, there will be days when you are in a rush, or feeling under pressure, and so allowing your baby to mess about (with the emphasis on 'mess') with her own spoon are too much to cope with. Aim to have two spoons on most occasions, nevertheless. It's all part of learning about food – your baby will be able to see what different food feels like if he's allowed to stir it and push it about with a spoon. When you first offer food on a spoon, you'll probably have to more or less tip the tiny quantities into your baby's mouth, emptying the spoon by inserting the edge of it and bringing it out against the top lip, so the contents are left behind. Sounds complicated, but it isn't and you'll do it more or less instinctively! Just remember to keep the amounts very small at first.

If you've left solids until six months or over, spoonfeeding isn't going to be a great feature of your life – it's so much simpler to offer finger food your baby can cope with herself. The temptation with spoonfeeding is to permit your idea of a sensible quantity to guide you, and not your baby's appetite. You keep spooning food in for as long as your baby lets you, and you may even try to squeeze in a few more spoonfuls on top. It has to be said that some babies really hate being spoonfed, and they only really start to enjoy solid food once they can feed themselves. Bear these

factors in mind and you'll go somewhere to stop mealtimes '
become a battle either now or in the second year.

SPROUTS (Brussels)

Brussels sprouts can be mashed or puréed and given as a second
stage vegetable. Small, tender sprouts make good finger food,
though you may have to chop them first as they may be too
'chewy'.

When? From the second stage of WEANING.

SQUASH

Fruit squash is not suitable for babies and small children, because
it contains artificial ADDITIVES AND COLOURINGS, as well as
sweeteners.

STEAMING

This is a cooking method that retains more of the nutrients in
food than boiling, though it does take longer. STERILISING
feeding equipment by steaming is becoming more popular.
You need to buy a purpose-made electrical unit, which costs
around £30.

STERILISING

If your baby is bottle fed or even if she only has the occasional
bottle, all the feeding equipment she uses each time must be as
clean as possible. This means you need to wash everything
thoroughly, and then rinse it, before sterilising by either:
i) immersing the items in a sterilising solution, which can be
either liquid, such as Milton, mixed with the appropriate amount
of water (see the instructions on the bottle of liquid) or tablets
(like Maws sterilising tablets) dissolved in water. This gives a
solution of sodium hyperchloride, which in a variable amount of
time according to the strength of the product used, kills bacteria
and which is considered harmless in itself. However, manufacturers now recommend rinsing off the residue of this chemical by
sluicing all the sterilised items in cooled, boiled water before

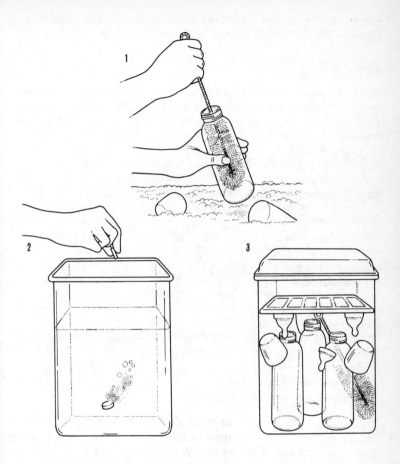

How to sterilise equipment in sterilising solution
1 Wash the equipment in soapy water, making sure that you remove any milk deposits inside bottles and teats. Rinse thoroughly.
2 Fill the sterilising tank with clean cold water. Add the sterilising solution or tablets, carefully following the instructions, and allow them to dissolve before adding the equipment.
3 Add the equipment and place a floating tray on top to keep everything submerged. Make sure there are no air bubbles as this will prevent parts of the equipment from being sterilised properly. Leave for as long as it states in the directions.

re-use, as this is safer for a baby than ingesting what remains of the solution. You need to mix up a fresh solution each day.

ii) boiling each item in a pan for 10 minutes.

iii) STEAMING each item in a special steam steriliser.
Overall, there's not much to choose between the different methods. You have to buy the sterilising liquid or tablets, and possibly a 'sterilising unit', though any sort of large plastic container would do. The advantage of the unit is that it is the right size to hold a number of bottles and teats, and you may get a sinker for the top of the container that makes sure all the items stay immersed without bobbing up and getting air in. Boiling obviously uses fuel, and the initial outlay for the steam steriliser is quite hefty – about £30 – though running costs are minimal. Leaving the items to be sterilised in a solution or a steamer is probably easier than making sure a pan doesn't boil dry, but boiling is very quick, especially if you only have the odd bottle to do, and there are no chemicals involved in boiling or steaming. In the end, it's up to you to decide what advantages and disadvantages are important to you and what you find most convenient.

Items that have been sterilised are safe as long as they are kept clean and dust free until the next use. Keep teats in a clean jam jar, and bottles with their covers on, until you need them again. Jugs used for mixing feeds, spoons (not metal if you use a sterilising solution), bottle tops, covers – everything used with the feed needs to be sterilised. Dummies should be sterilised once a day, and ideally a fresh one used if one falls on the ground. This isn't quite so vital as sterilising the bottle, however, (depending on where the dummy fell, of course) and washing well in running water should be sufficient if you don't have a sterilised one available. Milk deposits can collect round the neck of the dummy, even if your baby only brings back a little milk after or between feeds, so regular sterilising is important, as a rule. This is because the greatest risk of infection comes from milk traces; warm milk is a perfect breeding ground for bacteria, and bottle fed babies are at risk of GASTROENTERITIS if their bottles and other feeding equipment are not kept germ-free by sterilising. You should maintain the sterilising routine for as long as your baby gets milk from a bottle. Bowls, plates cups and spoons used with solid food don't need to be sterilised unless they're used with a very young baby under four months (who is probably too young for solids anyway . . .). Simply wash and rinse well.

STOOLS

The bowel motion. Those of a fully breastfed baby are daffodil-yellow, very soft and they don't smell offensive. A bottle fed baby has pale brown stools that may be more 'formed'. Some brands of formula milk cause greenish stools. However, as soon as your baby gets onto more than a small amount of foods other than milk his stools will start to change. It's not uncommon to see undigested food in your baby's stools. Beans, for instance, pass straight through without being digested in many babies of under a year.
See also CONSTIPATION; DIARRHOEA

STORING BREAST MILK

BREAST MILK is safe in the fridge for 24 hours, and it will keep in the freezer for three months or more. Store it however you like, a bottle isn't necessarily the most convenient way. A lidded plastic jug may be easiest while the milk's in the fridge. You can then pour it into a bottle when it needs to be used. You can freeze tiny amounts of it in ice cube trays, or in plastic lidded cups. As long as the storage item can be sterilised before you use it, and it won't smash at low temperatures, you can use it to store breast milk. Remember to leave a space in the container to allow for some expansion when the milk freezes.
See EXPRESSING BREAST MILK

STRAWBERRIES

See BERRIES

SUCKING REFLEX

The sucking reflex means a baby is able to draw the nipple into his mouth, put pressure on it with his jaws and tongue and thus

181

extract the breast milk in the breast. Although babies can and do suck while still in the uterus, the whole sucking/swallowing mechanism doesn't fully develop until about 36 weeks gestation, and so a PRE-TERM BABY may have difficulty in feeding for this reason.
See BREASTFEEDING

SUGAR

Sugar is a simple carbohydrate, and forms of it are found naturally in many foods. However, when sugar is added to foods in order to sweeten them (or sometimes to preserve them as well), the food is not nutritionally improved in any way. Taking in too much sugar over a long period of time can lead to overweight (because of the excess calories taken via the sugar), poor health, that addictive 'sweet tooth' and rotten teeth. Added sugar is almost always refined white sugar from sugar beet or sugar cane. Brown sugar – of whatever sort – sometimes has a very few extra minerals in it, but there's not a lot to choose between white and brown in terms of health. It's going to be difficult to stop your child enjoying sugary foods when he has them, but you can do a lot in this first year to stop the development of a sweet tooth, and to preserve the good healthy body nature gave him! There's a case for saying that we're almost programmed to enjoy sweet things – breast milk is actually quite sweet-tasting, and babies enjoy naturally sweet foods like apples, carrots and pears, but that's no reason to make things sweeter than they are in their unadulterated form. It's difficult to 'overdose' on the sugar in carrots – you'd have to eat several pounds. But it's easy to go through a lot of sugar when it's added by the spoonful to other foods.

If you're bottle feeding, never add sugar to the feed. If you offer water at any time (whether you're breast or bottle feeding) never sweeten it. First solids in particular should be sugar-free – many of the branded baby rices and other packet purées have sugar in them, so you need to read labels carefully. It may not be sucrose, but added glucose, fructose, maltose, dextrose are no better. In fact, there's no reason why your baby should have much added sugar at all even when he extends his range of solid foods. Keep sugar to a minimum by only using it occasionally to sweeten otherwise bitter foods (some stewed apple can be unpalatable without it, for instance) and often concentrated apple juice could be used instead. Don't get into a habit of sugaring your baby's breakfast cereal. If he needs medicines at any time, ask the doctor to prescribe a sugar-free version of whatever it is he needs, especially if the medicine is something he needs to take over a long period. Over-the-counter medicines such as paracetamol syrup can be usually bought in sugar-free brands, too. Avoid the introduction of sweets, biscuits and cakes, and sweet puddings, as far as you can.

SULTANAS

See RAISINS AND SULTANAS

SUPPER

If supper means a light meal taken just before going to bed, then your baby doesn't need anything more than a last milk feed, bottle or breast, in the first year. But supper can also mean TEA and it can be an important meal in the day.

SWEDE AND TURNIP

Mashed or puréed, swedes and turnips are naturally sweet and enjoyed by most babies. You do need to cook them fairly well in order to mash them sufficiently thoroughly.

When? From the first stage of WEANING.

SWEET POTATO

You can get sweet potatoes more easily than used to be the case – use them with your baby just as you would POTATO.

SWEETS

There is no reason why you can't delay sweets until well after your baby's a year old, although it's harder to do so in a family where there are older children who do eat sweets. With firstborn

183

children it's simple enough but you may have to explain gently to grandparents and others that sweets are not good for your baby, and you intend delaying their introduction as long as possible. Everyone is aware of the way that sugar spoils the appetite for more nourishing foods, rots the teeth and creates an unhealthy 'sweet tooth' – and sweets are virtually pure sugar. It's up to you whether you find a total sweet ban desirable or practical as your child gets older, and in any case, that question goes beyond the scope of this book. But banning them totally at this age does no harm at all socially and it may have benefits for the future.

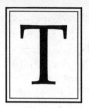

TEA*

At some time between six months and ten months, most babies are on three meals a day. Tea is one of them, at a time convenient to you and your baby. Five o'clock is a reasonable hour, as it gives you time to clear away before you need to start thinking about bedtime. However, if you prefer to eat as a family and you're not all in until after six, then your baby can fit in with this, too. He'll probably need some sort of snack and a milk drink sometime around three or four to keep going, though. Ideas for your baby's tea might include the ideas for LUNCH if tea is the main meal, or else: cheese on toast; scrambled egg; boiled egg; sandwiches; yoghurt and fresh fruit; mashed banana, with coconut sprinkled on top as an optional extra; short-grain rice pudding with raisins; pasta with cheese.

Tea as a drink is in no way suitable for a young baby.

TEATS

In the UK, teats are the rubber tops that fit onto a baby's feeding bottle, and nipples are the real thing on the mother's breast. In the US and in other English-speaking countries, the definitions are reversed – which must lead to at least the occasional bout of confusion at international conferences and elsewhere. To use the UK meaning of the word, teats come in different shapes and with different sized-holes. Usually, the larger a baby grows, the larger the teat hole he'll need (though you can enlarge an existing hole with a thick hot needle). Newborn teats usually have a small sized hole. Different liquids sometimes need different sized-holes – if you're using expressed breast milk or fruit juice, both of which are thinner than formula milk, a small hole may be sufficient. But, babies have different preferences and you may need to experiment. With repeated use and sterilisation, holes get too big, the rubber gets worn and sticky and the teat has to be discarded. You can choose between latex rubber and silicone rubber. Latex is soft and pliable, and many babies prefer it. However, silicone rubber lasts far longer, and if your baby is happy with it, its long life makes it more convenient.

If you're fully BOTTLE FEEDING, you'll need at least four teats on the go at any one time, so you always have a clean, sterilised one. Remember that STERILISING the teats between uses is essential for the first six months of your baby's life, and also beyond this age if the teats are used with milk. So-called orthodontic or natural teats, specially shaped with a flat or flattish top, are marketed as being better for a baby's jaw and dental development than the standard sort, and maybe that's true. Some normally breastfed babies do seem to feed better when given a bottle with an orthodontic teat. Don't be fooled by claims that these teats simulate a sucking action that's identical to the action used in breastfeeding, however. A breastfed baby uses his lips, gums, chin and tongue quite differently.

Concern has been expressed in various quarters about the safety of the rubber used in baby's teats and dummies. American safety standards have reduced the amount of chemical preservative permitted in teats and European standards have become more stringent, too. It could well be that the long-term hazards associated with feeding from a rubber teat, quite apart from the disadvantages to the baby who is *not* having breast milk, have yet to be fully documented.

TEETHING

Teething is the process whereby a baby's first teeth emerge and it can lead to painful gums. Breastfeeding babies occasionally find feeding causes discomfort, and if your baby starts refusing the breast for no obvious reason, and she's anything from three months old, it's just possible teething pain may be to blame (see BREAST REFUSAL). Teething gel applied to the gums just before a feed may help. Because a teething baby's saliva changes in acidity, you *may* find your NIPPLES become sore (though this is quite a rare cause of sore nipples because when sore nipples occur with an older baby it's more likely to be a result of

THRUSH). It will help to rinse your nipples after every feed with water, to wash away your baby's saliva. If your baby is going through a painful few days (and nights) with teething, it may not be a good idea to introduce new feeding experiences such as sitting in a high chair, finger food or new tastes and textures. She'll be happier and less fractious if you keep to the safe and familiar.

TEST WEIGHING

A breastfed baby is sometimes weighed immediately before and then immediately after a breastfeed, in order to ascertain just how much BREAST MILK has been taken. This is called 'test weighing'. The practice has just about nothing to be said in its favour. All authorities on breastfeeding speak with one voice on this and yet babies are still test weighed in many hospitals and baby clinics. There are a number of reasons why it is such an anxiety-making waste of time. Among them is the fact that all babies take different amounts of breast milk at each feed, partly because their appetite waxes and wanes throughout the day, and partly because mothers produce more at some times of the day than at others. So, if you test weigh once, it tells you nothing about the other feeds the baby may have in the next 24 hours. The feed you 'tested' may have been an unusually meagre one or an unusually generous one. You can't tell in advance how often that baby is going to feed in the next 24 hours, either.

Another reason is that we just don't know how much breast milk is needed for each individual baby. Attempts are made to standardise requirements, usually based on what we know of bottle fed babies' needs in terms of volume of milk compared to body weight of baby. But breast milk is different, and so are all babies. Your baby may not have 'standard' needs anyway – he may need more or less than the average, whatever that average is deemed to be. Test weighing won't enlighten you either way. Test weighing also puts pressure on mothers. A mum may want to breastfeed, and yet be told, or suspect herself, that because of her baby's weight, behaviour, appearance or whatever, she's not producing enough. This is enough to make her worried, and she then needs practical hints on increasing her MILK SUPPLY, or else reassurance, based on good quality information, that in fact she has sufficient milk. Feeding, while you know that the scales are waiting, willing your baby not to drop off to sleep too soon but to take as much as she can, and hoping that the test weight will prove she's had a 'good' feed, is enough to inhibit your LET-DOWN REFLEX anyway, and reduce the amount of milk available to your baby. Resist any suggestions that your baby should be test weighed, unless she has been ill or she was a PRE-TERM BABY, which might mean that the doctors need a precise indication of the volume of fluid taken at each feed. Test weighing should be seen as outmoded and discredited.

TEXTURE OF FOOD

Right from the start of WEANING, give your baby the chance to experience a variety of textures by preparing even identical foods in different ways – mashing roughly or smoothly, puréeing, mixing the food with something else to make it feel different in the mouth or chopping and slicing (for babies who can cope with this). Babies who usually have PURÉES or who only ever have commercial BABY FOODS can get very conservative about lumps.

THRUSH

Thrush is a fungal infection (also known as *Candida albicans*). It can affect warm, moist areas of the body, so in women, for example, the vagina is a favoured place. Babies can get thrush on their bottoms as a complication of nappy rash and in their mouths. It's not uncommon after a course of antibiotics, as the medicine kills off the bacteria that keep the fungus at bay. If your baby has thrush in her mouth and you're breastfeeding, you may get sore, itchy NIPPLES as the thrush gets passed on to you via your baby's mouth. Some babies find it uncomfortable to suck if they have thrush; more commonly it barely affects them, though if you look inside the mouth there may be white patches or a coating on the tongue. If you suspect thrush, see your doctor, and make sure both you and the baby are treated with the appropriate anti-fungal cream (for you) and drops (for the baby). A home remedy is to dissolve a teaspoonful of bicarbonate of soda in a cup of boiled, cooled water, and swab each nipple and the inside of your baby's mouth with cotton wool (clean cotton swab for each nipple and a fresh one for the mouth, of course).

TINNED FOODS

Tinned food which is not specifically designed for infants, can be used for babies under a year occasionally, as long as they don't contain SALT, SUGAR or artificial ADDITIVES AND COLOURINGS. If you don't use all the contents straightaway, store the remainder in the fridge having first put them into a cup or bowl. You need to do this because once in contact with the air, the metal of the can and of the material used to solder it together (possibly lead), starts to erode and traces of it seep into the food. Canned BABY FOODS are normally of a high standard and better for your baby than most other canned foods. However, bear in mind that good quality fresh food is always better than canned food for everyone, and especially your baby.

TOMATO

Your baby's first tomatoes should be peeled (the best way of peeling them is to slit the skins and then pour boiling water over them – the skins come away quite easily then). You can mash them and mix the pulp with something else, such as potato or pasta. When your baby's about ten months or so you can chop up whole tomatoes without peeling, although you could find the undigested skins in your baby's nappy! Bought tomato purée (unsalted) in small quantities can be used to flavour a meal for your baby. Commercial tomato ketchup isn't suitable for a baby as it is normally full of salt, sugar and highly spiced.

When? From the second stage of WEANING, (at first peeled, pipped and mashed).

TOO MUCH MILK

Some mothers feel they produce too much BREAST MILK. You may always feel uncomfortably full; you continue to leak copiously even after the first few weeks, when this has usually settled

189

down. Your baby may gasp and splutter at the breast, over-whelmed by the fast flow. This can be a problem, and in some cases, it's bothersome enough to make the whole business of breastfeeding messy and annoying all the time. It's often associated with BLOCKED DUCTS which are a problem in themselves. Feeding from one breast per feed, and not even offering the baby the second side (offering the unused side first next time) cuts down the stimulation of the supply and some women doing this find the problem ceases.

See LEAKING FROM BREASTS

TRAVEL

Very tiny babies aren't usually too much of a problem on a journey, as long as they're fed when they want to be fed and have a warm comfortable place to sleep. Older babies are less likely to sleep in a car, train or plane and you may find they are thirstier than normal. If your baby's on fluids other than milk, take along a good supply. Commercial BABY FOODS come in very useful on journeys, especially the ones in jars as all you need to take with you is the jar and a spoon (no can opener needed nor access to boiling water) to serve it directly to your baby. Babies who can cope with finger food may need occasional non-messy SNACKS to keep them happy between stops. You do need to be mindful of the risk of CHOKING though – your baby shouldn't eat in the back of the car if there is no adult apart from the driver to keep an eye on her.

See also HOLIDAYS

TURKEY

Use as CHICKEN in your baby's diet. Chopped up small, the turkey on the Christmas menu can be shared by a baby ready for the second stage of WEANING. Turkey, like chicken, is low in fat and it's a nutritious food for everyone, not just babies, and not just at Christmas.

TURNIP

See SWEDE AND TURNIP

TWINS

Twins are more likely than singletons to have feeding difficulties at birth, because they are more likely to be born pre-term or very small. You'll need encouragement and motivation to feed your twins if they aren't born at term, but of course it *can* be done (see PRE-TERM BABY). Full-term, average weight twins feed just like one baby twice over – and because your breasts are being stimulated twice as much, you'll produce twice as much milk (the same goes for triplets). It is the practical aspects of feeding twins and triplets which cause the problems rather than the physiological ones, by and large. Feeding two babies takes such a lot of time, though mothers of breastfeeding twins find very often that once the initial time-consuming weeks are over, breastfeeding is actually easier and quicker than bottle feeding could be. So it's worth persevering, and getting lots of help with other tasks such as washing and changing to allow you the time to feed and rest.

Some twin mothers combine breast and bottle feeding, because this way someone else can feed one baby while the other is at the breast. You can do this with formula milk or by EXPRESSING BREAST MILK. If you do it with formula, you need to realise that this will mean your breasts will produce less than the babies need to be fully breastfed, and that formula feeding has disadvantages of its own (see COMPLEMENTARY AND SUPPLEMENTARY BOTTLES). However, doing it this way may be your way of coping and the only way you can make sure that both twins get any of the benefits of breastfeeding. Learning to feed two babies at once is a useful skill, as it's a real time saver. It also means that the twin with the stronger suck (there's nearly always a difference) gets the LET-DOWN REFLEX working on one side, which usually means the milk starts to flow on the other as well, thereby encouraging the weaker twin to suck too. As your twins get older they may resist being fed in this way – fortunately by this time feeds are likely to be quicker anyway. When you start giving solids, two high chairs side-by-side, one bowl and one spoon seems to be the easiest way if you're spoonfeeding.

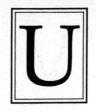

UNDERWEIGHT

See WEIGHT

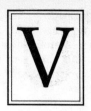

VEGANISM

People who are vegans don't eat any animal products at all, which means they don't have dairy products (such as milk or cheese) or eggs in their diet. Babies who are being brought up as vegans are at a nutritional disadvantage, as plant foods may not provide the calories and calcium growing babies and toddlers need. All vegans need to take a vitamin supplement of B12 in order to avoid anaemia. The disadvantages may be made up for by the fact that most vegans (like vegetarians) are knowledgable about food values, and can achieve an adequate diet with very careful thought. For more information, write to the Vegan Society.
See USEFUL ADDRESSES

VEGETABLES

In general, vegetables provide vitamins and minerals, and some contain a small amount of protein. Babies under a year need their vegetables cooked, on the whole, as their digestive system can't manage to fully metabolise the vegetables in their raw state – this may not actually harm your baby, but it does mean she's getting less than the full value out of her food. First vegetables, when your baby is just moving on to solids, can include carrots, potatoes, cauliflower, parsnips, turnips and swedes. Green leafy vegetables can come next.
See SPINACH; WEANING

VEGETARIANISM

It's perfectly possible for a child to be weaned on to a vegetarian diet and to grow up healthy – and it's easier for this to happen than if the child is introduced to VEGANISM. A vegetarian diet includes a ready source of good-quality protein of foods such as milk, cheese and eggs. If you are informed about healthy eating, and take care over what your child eats (as most vegetarians do, in my experience) then a meatless diet is unlikely to adversely affect your child's growth.

See USEFUL ADDRESSES

VITAMINS

Vitamins are substances found in foods; they are essential to life, and, so far as we know, human beings need 13 different vitamins in order to preserve health and growth. Vitamins have different functions, and one vitamin may have several properties. Some vitamins are easily lost in storage and in cooking. Milk for instance, is affected by light and loses some of its vitamin B2 content sitting on the doorstep (it would be better if milk bottles were made of darkened glass, in fact). Vitamin C can be found, among others, in vegetables and fruit, and this disappears into the cooking water when the food is heated – and if the food is kept hot for long after cooking the remaining vitamin C may be destroyed. Most food processing – canning, freezing, drying – affects the vitamin content. This doesn't mean that babies under a year should never have frozen, canned or dried food, but it does mean that your baby's diet shouldn't be based on food that's been processed in this way. A good supply of fresh foods is more likely to maintain the supply of vitamins he needs.

Babies on milk alone, breast or formula, don't normally need any supplementation of vitamins in the form of vitamin drops. Formula milk has had the required vitamins added to it, and breast milk contains all the vitamins a baby needs. It was thought at one time that breast milk was lacking in vitamin D and breastfed babies were routinely given vitamin drops. Further research has discovered that vitamin D is present in breast milk in both fat soluble and water soluble form, so there is indeed sufficient. Unless you yourself have a very poor diet, or are housebound for some reason and therefore unable to go out in daylight (the skin manufactures vitamin D after exposure to light), your breast milk will have the necessary vitamin D. If you do have a poor diet, or you are housebound, then you could ask your doctor about vitamin supplements for yourself.

When your baby is on mixed feeding, and he is on breast or formula milk and starts to build up a wide range of foods, his vitamin intake should really be sufficient. Current Department of Health advice is to give vitamin supplements in the form of vitamin drops after six months, however. It must be stated that by no means all experts accept that this sort of advice is necessary.

VOMITING

All young babies vomit to a certain extent – they may bring up a bit of milk with an after-feed burp, or simply allow the overflow to run out of the mouth because the stomach sends back the excess (and maybe more than just the excess) when it's full. This sort of vomiting is known as 'posseting'. If there's a largish amount of milk brought back, it may mean your baby feels hungry again quite quickly. You may have a 'SICKY' BABY who vomits a lot, before, during and after feeds. Make sure that you've had reassurance from the doctor or the health visitor that nothing serious is wrong. Projectile vomiting – when the vomit is habitually thrown out of the mouth with great force – is a symptom of PYLORIC STENOSIS and needs medical advice. Vomiting can also be a sign of illness, and if it goes on, or if it is combined with DIARRHOEA, fever, listlessness, excessive crying, or any other sign that makes you feel uneasy, then you need to ask your doctor's advice on what to do. There is a risk of DEHYDRATION in a young baby, especially.

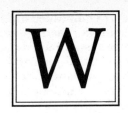

WATER

If you give your baby water it should be boiled and cooled first, for the first six months or so. This is a precaution, in order to make sure the water is pure. It's just possible that bacteria can be present especially if it's been standing in pipes, and boiling will reduce any risk. Water used for mixing formula milk feeds should be boiled first. After this age, it should be quite safe for your baby to have it straight from the tap, whether as a drink or to mix with something else. If you're on holiday abroad or anywhere you don't completely trust the water supply, buy bottled water. Make sure it's suitable for babies – the best way is to ask another mother if this is the case. Some bottled waters are carbonated, and some are naturally high in salts, and should be avoided. Sugar water (dextrose or glucose solutions) is sometimes given to new babies in hospital, yet it's been known for years that this is not necessary except in cases where the baby is unable to be breastfed, or is very ill because of low blood sugar. In fact, any fluid in these early days can interfere with the establishment of breastfeeding, so it shouldn't be given lightly.
See DRINKS

WEANING

Weaning is the gradual introduction of foods other than milk and we generally refer to these foods as 'solids', even though they may be anything but solid at first. Breastfeeding, or bottle feeding with baby formula milk, doesn't stop at the introduction of solids, in fact, it may go on for quite some time after.

So when should this gradual change start happening? Opinions and practices have differed, and will continue to do so, over the years and across generations and cultures. Current government advice in the UK is to introduce solids no earlier than three months and no later than six. There's normally no real need to introduce solids before four months at the earliest, however, and a baby who is feeding well and gaining weight satisfactorily is better off on milk alone for longer. If your baby's breastfed, remember it's agreed that BREAST MILK (from a reasonably-nourished mother) satisfies a baby's nutritional needs for at least the first four to six months. A few mothers breastfeed exclusively for longer than this, and if you remain well-nourished, and if your baby's happy and continuing to gain weight satisfactorily, this shouldn't present problems (see below). If your baby seems to need more than the breast milk you're giving her before she's reached four months of age, or if she's not gaining WEIGHT well, then feed her more often to increase your MILK SUPPLY. Even after four months, extra breast milk is still the best food to give her. There is nothing magical about the age of four months, or nothing especially valuable about getting your baby on to solids at this age. Go at your baby's pace – what may be the right age for one baby may be rather too soon for another.

Bottle fed babies generally start on solids earlier than breastfed babies. Whether this is because they 'signal' to their mothers they want something more or the mother is more easily disposed towards giving solids earlier, I don't know. In any case, as long as this isn't done before four months, it may be that a bottle fed baby is likely to need solids earlier than a breastfed one, although that viewpoint isn't reflected in the advice most often given to mothers, it has to be said. It's frequently assumed, in this context, that formula milk and breast milk are identical. They aren't, of course, though this assumption makes advice-giving easier. Unlike breast milk, formula milk doesn't change with the different needs of a growing baby, and as its composition is less perfectly suited to a baby's digestion, solids may be needed sooner. But, there's no reason to give your baby solids before six months if, again, he's happy and gaining weight satisfactorily on formula milk.

Giving solids early – before four months or before your baby is ready – has its problems. A young baby's delicate system can cope with breast milk or baby formula milk, but it can take time for her digestion to develop and be able to break down other substances. The problems that are caused aren't necessarily harmful in an obvious way, though some babies do become ill, and she may even appear to digest these early foods with reasonable success. But remember that solids, in all but the very smallest quantities, take the place of milk because they satisfy some of your baby's hunger. This doesn't matter in an older baby who needs to progress on to other foods anyway. But as breast milk (or in its absence, baby formula) is the ideal food for a young baby's growth and development, she may be getting less milk than she really needs for perfect nutrition. We know, too, that early solids can pre-dispose a baby to FOOD INTOLER-ANCE, and the inconvenience and, in severe cases, pain and discomfort this leads to makes early solids a quite unnecessary risk. If you have ALLERGY in your family, then early solids are even more ill-advised. Just occasionally, it might be advisable for a baby to be put on solids earlier than four months. It could be that a paediatrician has diagnosed an allergy to baby formula, and switching to another formula doesn't relieve the symptoms. RELACTATION is rarely suggested in these cases, but when it's possible, it is far better than going onto early solids, although of course the baby mustn't be allowed to go short of nourishment while the milk supply is being built up (see CHANGING: FROM BOTTLE TO BREAST). Too often, though, solids are suggested when there's a persistently low weight gain, without the mother being given any advice on increasing her milk supply (if she's breastfeeding), and without the baby being investigated for some underlying disorder or allergy. Mothers are told to give solids to help the baby sleep at night, or to settle him in the evening. Solids may encourage sleep (because of the 'full-up feeling'), or they may not. The problem is that most babies don't actually *need* foods other than milk at an early age. And if a baby's breastfed, early solids work like COMPLEMENTARY AND SUP-PLEMENTARY BOTTLES to undermine breastfeeding.

Don't feel too guilty if you want to introduce something else before your baby actually seems to need it (with the proviso, above, that you don't do it too soon). For instance, if your baby's breastfed, knowing she'll take a few spoons of something other than milk can be helpful if you have to leave her with a babysitter, or if you're going back to work. And some mothers want to introduce something of a routine into their baby's still-disordered life! Mixed feeding allows you to work towards this, too, as you can aim more precisely at an eventual basis of three meals a day.

By six months, most babies are at least starting to be weaned. It's been thought that a baby's iron stores begin to run down then, and so need supplementing with other foods. However, breastfed babies do get a small amount of iron in breast milk – more than it was previously thought – and older babies of healthy mums who are still exclusively breastfed may be perfectly healthy. Present knowledge isn't yet clear, however, and most experts in this area would suggest you start your baby on a few new tastes by six months. This means taking the initiative yourself if your baby hasn't dropped any hints by restless behaviour or a lack of weight gain or by showing an interest in what other people are eating. First tastes of new foods should be given in the tiniest quantities, off the very end of a spoon (see SPOONS AND SPOONFEEDING). Too much at once and your baby will simply allow it all to spill out. Don't expect to give more than a teaspoonful per session at first; you're just getting him used to different tastes and textures at this stage, with a view to building up slowly as you go along. It's up to you and your baby to choose the best time of day to give these early tastes, and it's probably easiest to think about what you'll want your eventual routine to be in terms of breakfast, lunch and tea or supper. After all, your baby will end up having three solid meals a day. It makes sense to aim at giving the first solids at a time which will approximate to one of these meals.

At first, give your baby her milk feed, or part of it, to start with, and this will take the edge off her hunger and keep her temper sweet! For breastfed babies, this might mean 'sandwiching' the solids between two 'sides'; for bottle fed babies, you can spoon-feed when the bottle's half finished or when you'd normally stop in order to wind your baby. It doesn't matter if you give the whole milk feed first, though, if that's what turns out to be easiest, as long as your baby doesn't fall asleep before you get round to giving the solids. As your baby gets older, it's perfectly alright to give the solids first, but the younger she is the more important milk is to her diet. Good first foods include rice and puréed fruit and vegetables. RICE is an ideal first cereal as it contains no GLUTEN. You can mix the cereal with expressed breast milk, your baby's usual baby formula or plain boiled water. Mashed banana – which most babies absolutely adore – is excellent, especially as you can vary the texture as your baby gets better at coping with lumps. The same goes for boiled, mashed potato.

What I have termed the 'first stage of weaning' throughout this book describes the period when you'll introduce the most easily-digested foods, and when milk will still form the basis of your baby's diet. First stage foods (suitable from a minimum age of four months) include rice, potatoes, carrots, cauliflower, turnips, leeks, apples, peaches, apricots, pears and bananas. The 'second stage of weaning' comes after your baby is used to three or four items from this first list, and is at least five months old. She can progress on to oats, barley, other green vegetables, other non-citrus fruits and meat. When the second stage of weaning is established, you can introduce other foods including wheat, citrus fruits, egg (first yolk, then white) and mild cheeses, if your baby is at least six months old. Even if you don't start weaning until six months, it's still sensible to begin with first stage-type foods and build up your baby's range gradually. These are merely guidelines, however, as no one can give you a blueprint of the perfect weaning order. There is no universally agreed sequence of foods, and although it seems fairly certain that some foods are more likely than others to be linked with food intolerance, there are grey areas in this whole field of study at present. For a table detailing one suggested order of foods, see page 201.

What about commercial BABY FOODS? They are used by almost everyone at some time, and they've much improved over the last few years. It is important to make sure you incorporate different textures right from the start, puréeing, mashing and then chopping as your baby gets more able to cope. Otherwise, you might have a bit of a problem getting her off smooth textures and on to your food. Babies enjoy FINGER FOOD too – foods like toast, chunks of apple or vegetable they can hold and suck or chew on (though you'll need to stay close by to help your baby if she bites off more than she can chew, literally). You should wait until your baby's well-established on solids before giving her foods high in fibre (like peas, beans and other pulses) and hard cheese. The reason for this is that these foods are hard to break down, and are therefore poorly digested.

Whenever you're introducing new foods, do so one at a time. If you're giving your baby cabbage for the first time, for instance, either give it on its own, or mixed with something your baby is used to, such as potato. In this way, if you get a reaction to the food, you can be sure to pinpoint which it is. And also don't SALT your baby's food. She can have more of what you're having to eat the older she gets – but if you're having a casserole or vegetables, leave the salt out until after the dish is cooked and you have removed your baby's portion.

Don't be in a hurry to cut down on the milk in your baby's diet, ideally, it should be a major part of her food intake for at least the first nine months to a year. Many babies go on breastfeeding after this age, and many babies still have bottles, too, though almost all are capable of learning to manage a spouted cup from about six months as well (see FORMULA MILK; MILK).

Weaning chart

Note: these are guidelines to help you and your baby make a gradual move from milk-only to family meals. It's not a blueprint – so be prepared to be flexible according to your individual baby's rate of progress, his physical needs and his likes and dislikes. Remember, you don't have to introduce other foods at four to five months: in fact, if your baby is happy on milk alone, and you're happy to go on feeding him exclusively on breast or formula milk, there's no reason to give him anything else.

		1st stage							
age in months	0–4	4–5	5–6	6–7	7–8	8–9	9–10	10–11	11–12
			2nd stage						
apple		=====							
apricot		=====							
aubergine		=====							
avocado			=====						
beans & pulses			=====						
beef			=====						
beetroot			=====						
berries			=====						
bread			=====						
broccoli			=====						

	age in months	0–4	4–5	1st stage 5–6	6–7 2nd stage	7–8	8–9	9–10	10–11	11–12
butter				=====						
cabbage				=====						
carrots			=====							
cauliflower			=====							
celery				=====						
cheese (soft, low fat)				=====						
cheese (hard)						==				
cherries				=====						
chicken				=====						
courgettes				=====						
cream				=====						
eggs (yolk)				=====						
eggs (white)					=====					
fish				=====						
grapefruit				=====						
grapes (peeled, pipped)				=====						
jams, spreads				=====						
lamb				=====						
leeks			=====							
lettuce							==			
liver (lamb's first)				=====						
margarine			=====							
mangoes			=====							
melon			=====							
milk (full-fat pasteurised milk)					=====					
mushrooms			=====							
nuts (ground)				=====						
oats				=====						
onion				=====						

(in small quantities for mixing only; if used as a drink, boil and dilute at first. Breast or formula is best for first 12 months)

age in months	0–4	4–5	5–6	6–7	7–8	8–9	9–10	10–11	11–12
			2nd stage						
oranges			=====	=====					
parsnips		=====	=====						
pasta			=====	=====					
pastry			=====	=====					
peaches			=====	=====					
peanut butter			=====	=====					
pears		=====	=====						
peas			=====	=====					
peppers			=====	=====					
pineapple			=====	=====					
plums			=====	=====					
pork (after lamb, chicken)			=====	=====					
potato (mashed)		=====	=====						
potato (fried, roast occasionally)						==			
rhubarb				==					
rice		=====	=====						
salads						==			
seeds			=====	=====					
sharon fruit			=====	=====					
spinach				==					
sprouts (Brussels)			=====	=====					
sprouts (bean)			=====	=====					
swede, turnip		=====	=====						
tomatoes (peeled, seeded)			=====	=====					
turkey			=====	=====					
wheat			=====	=====					
yeast extract								===	
yoghurt			====						

Weaning: from breast or bottle The 'other' meaning of weaning . . . this refers to the period during which a baby makes the change to getting all of his drinks from a cup, as opposed to a bottle or the breast. Because both bottles and breasts are sources of comfort for a baby, the change is a developmental and even a social one as well as being nutritionally important. Most babies actively enjoy sucking, and the time they're actually ready to give it up of their own accord varies. The majority of them will be happy enough to start taking at least some of their drinks from a spouted cup at some time between the ages of five and nine months.

If you're keen for your baby *not* to have any bottles, or to have stopped breastfeeding completely, before, say, 18 months or so, then it's a good idea to take active measures before the age of a year. Many babies do give up the breast or bottle by themselves before this, or before 18 months, but you can't guarantee it. Active measures may include: wheeling your baby out in the pushchair or pram to allow her to drop off without a 'sucking feed'; distracting her with an amusing game or activity at a time she'd normally expect to suck; stopping her from falling asleep in the middle of her breast or bottle; making sure you're away from the place she normally feeds in, perhaps out of doors; always giving her meals in a high chair and never on your lap; making feeds shorter; making the change from always putting her to bed yourself (which will make her think of a breastfeed, if you're breastfeeding) and giving the task to another familiar and loved person. You'll no doubt be able to think of other wiles which will fit in with what you know of your baby's personality and needs, and which will avoid any unhappiness on her part. The easiest way to wean, both physically (if you're breastfeeding) and emotionally, is gradually. Don't feel you have to wean, of course. Many babies have bottles well into toddlerhood and beyond, and mothers who breastfeed for as long as this aren't a rarity at all, either. (The only difficulty might be with a toddler taking a lot of milk via a bottle every day and so his milk intake prevents him being hungry for a wider range of solid foods.) If you want to leave it up to your baby to organise, then do so!

WEIGHT

Because weight is an easily measured indicator of a baby's health and development, babies are routinely weighed at birth and at intervals thereafter. It's normal for babies to lose up to ten per cent of their birthweight in the first days after birth, although some babies, especially those who feed strongly, often from day one, lose virtually nothing. Some babies regain all that lost weight within a week; while others can take two to three weeks, or even more. On average, a new baby gains between four and eight ounces per week in the first month, and thereafter between six and eight ounces until the age of five months, when the rate of weight gain starts to slow down to about four ounces a week. Babies older than this will gain less, and by the end of the first year, your baby is probably only putting on about two ounces a week. However, working on weekly averages like this is potentially misleading although most people working in child-care, such as health visitors and midwives, use these guidelines as a rough rule of thumb in assessing a baby's progress. Some babies have a very erratic rate of weight gain; some weeks they may not gain anything at all, and other weeks they may put on a great deal. This can be especially true of exclusively breastfed babies, who are less likely to gain in a regular way. At your clinic, your baby's weight should be plotted on a graph and you can then see much more readily what his weight is doing.

A baby who weighed a fairly average seven pounds or so at birth, should weigh a fairly average 14 pounds at the age of four months, and a fairly average 21 pounds at a year. If your baby departs from his expected rate of weight gain, and continues to do so over a matter of weeks, then it doesn't necessarily mean that anything is wrong. Whatever, ask your health visitor how often she'd like to see you and your baby in order to weigh her. Once a fortnight is usually considered enough in the first three or four months and less often thereafter, though if you have older children, or a long distance to go to the clinic, you may not make it as regularly as this. A baby who's had feeding difficulties may need to be weighed weekly, and those who are slow to regain their birthweight may need even more frequent checking.

As mothers, we can't help having a tendency to focus on weight gain as the main symbol of our baby's progress. After all, it's just about the only thing you can actually measure, especially if you're breastfeeding. Factors like skin tone, brightness of eyes, alertness, contentedness, general health, normality of development and muscle tone are that much more difficult to assess unless you are especially trained. And a satisfactory weight gain is something that can come as a tremendous morale-booster if you're breastfeeding – you have the proof that your baby's 'getting enough', and that it's all your own work! But do remember that it is only one indication of your baby's well-being. A poor weight gain in itself should never be used as a reason for introducing bottles to a breastfed baby, unless there is clear evidence of a failure to thrive and efforts to increase the MILK SUPPLY have failed (see COMPLEMENTARY AND SUPPLEMENTARY BOTTLES).

Underweight   Lack of a satisfactory weight gain is very worrying. It may mean your baby is not feeding often enough, or not taking enough milk at each feed; it may mean she has some underlying disorder that's not allowing her to digest her food properly; if you're breastfeeding your MILK SUPPLY may not be enough; if you're bottle feeding your baby may be allergic to the formula you're using; your baby may be ill. On the other hand, she may just be a naturally slow gainer and perfectly healthy in all respects. Weight is only one indication of a baby's health in any case, but check with a health visitor or doctor. It may be that you need to increase your baby's food intake by increasing your milk supply if you're breastfeeding, or by increasing the number and/or volume of bottles. If your baby is over six months, introduce or increase the amount of solids (see WEANING).

Overweight   Overweight is not so much of a problem and time was when babies had to be round and fat in order to be considered 'bonny'. The practice of artificial feeding with high-sugar, high-fat milks and early solids given in a bottle allowed babies to put on more weight than they would otherwise have done. There are experts who feel that this excess weight in infancy leads in many cases to the risk of excess weight in childhood and adulthood. The prevailing ideas on ideal size have changed, now. Take a look at babies born in the 1950s (like me, for instance!), a goodly proportion of them are little Michelin men compared with babies today. This emphasis on slimness must be at least partly a good thing, given what we know about over-weight and its attendant health risks, not to mention the ridicule at school if the overweight baby becomes a tubby child. But the other side of the coin is that mothers now worry if their babies aren't slim enough. Babies who gain weight at a greater rate than the average raise eyebrows at baby clinics, and mothers are embarrassed if their babies look plumper than their peers.

The current state of knowledge is that if a baby is gaining a lot of weight on breast milk alone, then you don't need to be too concerned. Feed him according to appetite, and don't use his hunger as a reason for introducing solids early. Solids may increase his calorie intake, not lessen it. When the time comes to go onto mixed feeding, bear his appetite in mind and simply be extra sure to offer a healthy, low-sugar diet. Breastfed babies who seem 'overweight' almost always lose it once they're on the move, crawling and walking. If your baby's bottle fed, or on solids with bottles, and you're told he's overweight by your doctor or health visitor, then you need to intervene a little more directly. It is easy to overfeed a bottle fed baby, and it's possible he's having one bottle of milk (or two) more than he actually needs. Older babies on mixed feeding who are drinking a lot of ordinary full-fat pasteurised milk in a bottle may appear over-weight, this should be thought of as a food rather than a drink at this age, and it's high in calories. In both cases, offer water instead of milk, or offer the milk in a cup (to babies over five months) instead of a bottle. However, if you're mixing his feeds correctly, and not adding cereal to the bottle or over-doing the solids, then your bottle fed baby may simply be a 'good gainer', and will lose his 'extra' with increasing mobility. Babies up to a year are more amenable to changes in their diet than they are later. If you feel your baby's taking too much bottle milk, it's comparatively easy to alter this now, rather than facing the determination of toddlerhood!

WET-NURSING

Wet nursing is the practice of breastfeeding a baby who is not the mother's own. It used to be quite normal in previous centuries, when the baby's own mother had died or was unwilling to breastfeed. These days, it probably goes on in a casual way a lot more often than you might think, although it's more likely to be an arrangement that people fall into, rather than one they deliberately engineer. For example, a breastfeeding mother may be babysitting for a friend whose absence from the house is unexpectedly prolonged. The baby eventually cries from hunger and the babysitter may breastfeed him as being the most effective way of comforting him. On the other hand, it's also true that a few working mothers have sought out a breastfeeding childminder willing to feed their baby, too. It's a measure of the way this society regards breastfeeding that many people might think wet-nursing is a peculiar aberration, yet it's surely a better alternative to giving bottles or early solids. Although, it is true that many women could feel distressed at another woman having this sort of very special relationship with their child – and that's understandable.

WHO CODE

This is the World Health Organisation's code on the marketing and distribution of baby foods – that is, breast milk substitutes or FORMULA MILK. In 1981, the WHO endorsed a code which, for the first time, placed formal restrictions on the manufacturers of baby formula, and their agents. Recognising that this is an important child health issue, and one on which mothers need to have information rather than commercially-backed promotions, many nations campaigned to have the WHO code adopted by their own governments. In the UK a considerably weaker, watered down and fudged code was adopted known as the Food Manufacturers Federation Code. This, for example, outlaws the advertising of formula milk in the consumer press (that is, magazines bought from the news stand), yet it permits the advertising of bottles and teats in these same publications. And formula milk itself can be advertised in the 'mothercraft' books and magazines that mothers obtain direct from the health clinic.
See BREASTFEEDING; USEFUL ADDRESSES

WIND

Everybody takes in air – 'wind' – when they eat, but it does seem that babies are bothered by it, especially when they're young. The fact that it doesn't seem to be a problem with older babies

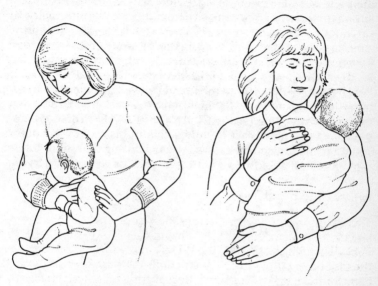

A good way to wind a baby is to sit him up on your lap, supporting his chest and leaning him forward slightly, then gently rub or pat his back with your other hand. Alternatively, lift him up against your chest so that his head can rest on your shoulder, and rub his back. You only need to do this for a few minutes.

may have something to do with the fact that the digestive system matures and becomes better able to handle wind. It may also be a result of the way we tend to have our babies lying flat for much of the time. Perhaps wind has less chance to escape this way. Babies in other cultures are sometimes carried upright against their mothers' bodies, and this posture may have something to do with the way wind isn't a problem. It's certainly the case that mothers of babies who cry a lot report that a baby sling which keeps the baby close to them is helpful. Of course, it's difficult to know where wind ends and distress at separation and loneliness begins. Parents often say that their baby sleeps between feeds if he's been given the chance to let out a large belch of air after his

209

breast or bottle feed. Restlessness and refusal to suck are often signs that your baby needs propping up to burp in mid-feed, too. All this is trial and error, and it depends on what sort of a baby you have. I do feel that some babies are windier than others, and you do need to respond to this need for deliberate 'winding'. However, some babies fall asleep or at any rate become very settled and soothed on the breast (or the bottle), and to wake them up to rub their backs in order to encourage the wind to come up can well and truly unsettle them and prevent a contented sleep.

Certain foods in your diet may seem to affect your baby when you're breastfeeding (see DIET AND BREASTFEEDING). Later on, your baby may react to new solids in his diet by apparent tummy pains, caused by gasses released during digestion. If this happens, then avoid this food for a week or two before trying again.

See also COLIC; CRYING

WOOLWICH SHELLS

Woolwich Shells is a brand name.
See BREAST SHELLS

WORKING

Whether or not you go back to work, and when you go back to work, after you have had your baby is a matter of choice and circumstance. If you return when the baby is still being breastfed, you may be able to continue breastfeeding, partially or fully. It's been known for mothers to go back as early as a few weeks after the birth, and EXPRESSING BREAST MILK during the working day and at home for the minder or nanny to give in a bottle. When a mother in this position is at home in the evenings and at weekends, she just feeds the baby as normal. It has to be said that this sort of regime needs a lot of motivation, plus the sort of working conditions that allow you to express in private, and to store the expressed milk hygienically. A fridge at work is essential, plus a cool-box for getting the milk from work to home unless you live very close.

If you decide that keeping up exclusive breastfeeding requires too high a price – after all, it's demanding, and working while your baby is small is demanding in itself – then you could consider breastfeeding when you're with your baby, and leaving formula milk for her when you're not. Doing this before your baby is two months old or so could mean that your breasts don't get the sort of stimulation they need to maintain a good MILK SUPPLY . . . it depends on how often you breastfeed, how well established your breast milk supply is and whether your baby is happy to have breast and bottle. If you continue to breastfeed frequently at weekends, you may have to express to keep yourself comfortable in the middle of the day at work. In practice, it seems to be the case that babies learn quite quickly that mum supplies the breast milk, and when someone else always gives the formula when mum isn't around, the baby is less likely to develop a preference for the bottle. If you're worried about going back to work because you feel, on the contrary, that your baby will never take to the bottle (and you've had a few failed attempts at it), don't be too anxious. Experiment with a larger-holed teat, don't be around when the bottle is given and accept that your baby won't starve herself. When it comes to the crunch, if she's hungry while you're away, she will eventually take something, even if her minder has to spoon the milk in. Babies already on solids are an easier proposition as they may be old enough to use a spouted cup for milk drinks in addition to the solid part of the meal.

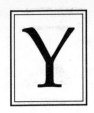

YEAST EXTRACT

Marmite is a yeast extract, and this popular savoury spread is rich in B vitamins and better for your baby than sweetened jams and spreads. However, because it has salt in it, you should only use tiny amounts when giving it to your baby. The taste is strong enough, and the texture spreadable enough, for small quantities to be quite sufficient anyway. You can add Marmite to soups and stews as well for flavour, and for its nutritional quality.

When? Towards the end of the first year only.

YOGHURT*

Once your baby is six months old or so, and able to take milk apart from breast milk or baby formula, you can give him yoghurt. Most yoghurt is based on COW'S MILK, but because lactic acid bacteria in the yoghurt partially digest the LACTOSE (milk sugar) in the milk, it's actually easier than straight cow's milk for a baby to digest. Whole milk yoghurt has a higher vitamin content than yoghurt made from skimmed or semi-skimmed milk, and as such, is more nutritious. However, you won't be using yoghurt as a substitute for milk in your baby's diet, so this factor isn't important. The best yoghurt for a child under one is natural and unsweetened. You can buy this sort in most supermarkets, with or without fruit. You can add your own fruit to plain yoghurt and serve that to your baby as well. Home-made yoghurt is easiest and more consistently successful with a yoghurt maker in my experience, but some people get good results with insulated biscuit tins or vacuum flasks.

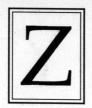

ZINC

A trace element in foods, zinc is one of several needed by the body in small but vital quantities for growth and health. Some years ago, zinc-deficient baby formula milk was found to contribute to skin, growth and developmental problems. It's now included in formula milk in higher quantities.

RECIPES

Apricot pudding
Avocado and yoghurt
Baby rice
Baked potato and vegetables
Banana and apple crumble
Beef casserole
Biscuits
Broccoli
Cabbage
Cake – sugar-free
Carrots
Casseroled beans
Cauliflower cheese
Cheese fingers
Cheesy celery
Cheesy potato
Coddled egg
Egg and tomato
Fish cakes
Fruit delight
Hot pot
Ice Cream
Jelly

Kidney and carrot
Leek broth
Liver
Meat loaf
Millet porridge
Muesli
Nectarine or peach pudding
Nut loaf
Oats and pear
Pancakes
Pasta and vegetable sauce
Plum pudding
Rice, chicken and cabbage
Risotto
Rusks
Sesame fingers
Soup
Spreads
Stewed apple
Stock for babies
Summer cup
Wholemeal bread
Yoghurt

APRICOT PUDDING

150g (6oz) apricots (peeled, chopped and stoned)
3 slices fresh or canned pineapple (choose the sort canned without syrup)
small amount of apple juice
3 tbsp natural yoghurt

Blend apricots with pineapple, apple juice and yoghurt.

Note: for a change try using fromage frais – a pleasant tasting, low-fat cheese – instead of yoghurt.

AVOCADO AND YOGHURT

Mash the flesh of half a ripe avocado with about 3 tbsp natural yoghurt.

BABY RICE – home made

Brown rice: mix 1 tbsp ground brown rice with 125ml ($\frac{1}{4}$ pint) of water, milk or a combination. Simmer for 5 minutes, stirring.
White rice: as above, using white rice or rice flakes.

BAKED POTATO AND VEGETABLES

1 medium potato (scrubbed)
2 tbsp mixed vegetables (from a freezer pack eg carrot and sweetcorn, peas and carrots etc)

Bake potato in oven, 180°C, 350°F, gas 4, until it feels soft when squeezed (about one hour). Cook vegetables. Scoop out potato flesh and mix with vegetables.

Note: a little grated cheese could be added to the potato flesh. This dish is more worthwhile if you are already cooking baked potatoes for the rest of the family. Otherwise, mash boiled potato.

BANANA AND APPLE CRUMBLE

2 bananas (sliced)
1 dessert apple (peeled, cored and sliced)

Topping:
100g (4oz) wholemeal flour
50g (2oz) butter or margarine
1 tbsp sultanas

Mix fruit and place in small ovenproof dish. Rub fat into flour and add sultanas and place on top of fruit. Cook at 190°C, 375°F, gas 5, for 20 minutes.

Note: this quantity would serve four, or two adults and one baby.

215

BEEF CASSEROLE

1 tbsp sunflower oil
200g (8oz) stewing steak (trimmed and cubed)
1 medium onion (chopped finely)
1 small swede (peeled and chopped)
1 large carrot (peeled and chopped)
1 tbsp tomato purée
50g (2oz) broccoli (chopped)
275ml (½ pint) water (approximately)
bouquet garni

Fry meat and onion in oil for 2 minutes. Add vegetables (apart from broccoli) and mix. Add tomato purée. Transfer to ovenproof dish, add bouquet garni and water and cook at 170°C, 325°F, gas 3, for 1½–2 hours, adding broccoli half an hour before the end of cooking.

Note: this quantity would serve two adults and a baby.

NUTTY BISCUITS

50g (2oz) wholemeal flour (plain or self-raising)
50g (2oz) ground nuts (eg hazelnuts, unsalted peanuts, almonds)
50g (2oz) butter or margarine
1 egg (beaten)
25g (1oz) raisins

Rub fat into flour. Add remaining ingredients and mix to a dough. Roll out to 50mm (¼ inch). Cut into round shapes with a biscuit cutter to make 12–15 biscuits. Bake at 190°C, 375°F, gas 5, for 15 minutes.

Note: self-raising flour gives a more spongy texture – and if you use it, prick your biscuits with a fork before baking.

BROCCOLI

1–2 sprigs broccoli (washed)

Bring 250ml (½ pint) water to the boil and add broccoli. Simmer for 5 minutes. Drain, mash and sieve.

Note: avoid the tough stems of broccoli.

CABBAGE

2 leaves crisp white cabbage

Shred finely and put into a very small amount of water. Bring to boil and simmer with lid on pan for 10 minutes. Drain and chop to the texture your baby prefers.

Note: steaming will preserve more nutrients. Takes about 20 minutes.

SUGAR-FREE CAKE

300g (12oz) pineapple (tinned in natural juice or fresh)
450g (1lb) sultanas (washed well and dried)
2 tbsp apple juice
2 eggs (beaten)
4 tsp baking powder
200g (8oz) wholemeal flour
50g (2oz) butter or margarine

Blend or liquidise pineapple. Mix with sultanas and fruit juice. Leave to stand for about one hour. Add beaten eggs and baking powder to the fruit mixture. Rub fat into flour and add this to fruit and eggs. Place in greased, lined tin and bake at 190°C, 375°F, gas 5, for 75–90 minutes.

Note: although this cake has no sugar, it is still high in sweetness and calories because of the dried fruit. It has a high fibre content, too, and babies and toddlers should only be given small pieces at a time.

BABY'S CARROTS

2 small carrots (scrubbed if new, peeled if old, and chopped)
enough chicken stock to blend

Steam the carrots and blend with the stock.

CASSEROLED BEANS

1 cup beans or pulses (cooked)
1 tomato (peeled)
2 dtsp oat flakes
1 egg (beaten)

Mash beans (or put in food processor) with tomato, oats and egg. Put into an oiled casserole, with a lid, and bake at 180°C, 350°F, gas 4, for 30 minutes.

Note: to cook beans, soak overnight in cold water and then bring to boil and simmer, 45 minutes for haricot beans, 60 minutes for butter beans.

CAULIFLOWER CHEESE

4–5 small florets cauliflower
1 tbsp baby rice or ground rice
4 tbsp milk
25g (1oz) cheese (grated)

Cook cauliflower florets until tender in a small amount of water (approximately 5 minutes). Drain and reserve water. Mix reserved water with rice and sufficient milk to give a thick sauce. Heat sauce in a pan for 5 minutes, stirring. Remove from heat and add cheese. Add chopped cauliflower and serve.

CHEESE FINGERS

100g (4oz) wholemeal self-raising flour
50g (2oz) butter or margarine
1 egg (beaten)
50g (2oz) finely grated hard cheese (eg cheddar)
25g (1oz) ground nuts (eg hazelnuts, unsalted peanuts)
pinch salt

Sieve flour, add nuts and salt, rub in fat. Stir in cheese and add egg to make a dough. Knead and roll out to 50mm (¼ inch) thickness. Cut into finger shapes. Bake at 190°C, 375°F, gas 5, for 10–15 minutes.

Note: this quantity makes about 40 fingers. They freeze well.

CHEESY CELERY

2 stalks celery
1 dtsp ground rice
125ml ($\frac{1}{4}$ pint) milk (approximately)
25g (1oz) grated low fat cheese (eg Edam)

Steam the celery. Mix milk with ground rice and boil to thicken. Add cheese to sauce and pour over celery.

CHEESY POTATO

2 small potatoes (scrubbed)
1 small egg (beaten)
2 tbsp milk
2 tbsp cheese (grated)

Boil potatoes until tender, remove skin. Mash with egg and enough milk to give a soft consistency. Add half the cheese. Place in small ovenproof dish and sprinkle over the rest of the cheese. Bake at 190°C, 375°F, gas 5, 15–20 minutes.

Note: half quantities would be enough for younger babies.

CODDLED EGG

Bring a medium egg to the boil in a small pan. Remove from the heat. Cover the pan and leave for 7 minutes. Shell and mash.

Note: this is a good way to introduce egg white to a baby, as the slow cooking makes it more digestible.

BABY'S EGG AND TOMATO

Scramble an egg with a little milk and add to half a skinned tomato, de-seeded. Add a little finely chopped parsley.

BABY'S FISH CAKES

250g (½lb) white fish
250g (½lb) potato
wholemeal breadcrumbs
small egg (beaten)
chopped parsley

Cook potatoes, and while doing so steam the skinned fish on an oven-proof plate on top of the pan for 10 minutes. Fish is cooked when the flakes separate easily. Drain potatoes thoroughly and mash or sieve. Drain fish (reserving liquid); flake and check very carefully for bones. Mix fish with potato and parsley. Shape into 6–8 cakes and coat with egg and breadcrumbs, place on a baking tray and cook at 180°C, 350°F, gas 4, for 20–30 minutes until hot and crispy.

Note: the reserved fish juices can be used as the basis for a sauce.

FRUIT DELIGHT

1 banana
1 Comice pear
1 dessert apple
1 tsp apple juice

Peel and chop fruit, coring the pear and apple. Blend ingredients together.

Note: half these quantities would be all that was needed for a young baby. Freeze the remainder.

HOT POT

100g (4oz) stewing lamb (trim fat and cut into small pieces)
2 medium potatoes (sliced thinly)
½ small onion (chopped finely)

Layer the ingredients in a casserole dish, finishing with potato. Add enough water to come halfway up the mixture. Stew on stove top by boiling, and then simmering with a lid on for 1½ hours, *or* casserole in the centre of the oven for 2½–3 hours at 190°C, 375°F, gas 5.

Note: depending on the age and appetite of your baby, this will make two or three portions. Freeze the remainder.

ICE CREAM

275ml (½ pint) single cream
275ml (½ pint) whole milk
2 eggs
1 vanilla pod
6 dtsp clear honey

Simmer milk with vanilla pod for 5 minutes. Allow to cool a little. Beat eggs, sieve into milk. Cook very gently for 10–15 minutes until mixture is thick enough to coat the back of a spoon. Remove from heat. Mix honey with cream and add to milk mixture. Freeze. After 2 hours remove from freezer and beat. Freeze a further two hours or until set.

Note: though this is more nutritious than bought ice cream on the whole, it is still sweet and high in fat, so small portions only for babies and toddlers.

FRUIT JELLY

1 tsp powdered gelatine
4 tbsp fruit juice (fresh or carton eg orange, blackcurrant, apple)

Dissolve gelatine in 4 tbsp hot (not boiling) water. Stir in fruit juice. Leave to set in fridge for approximately 45 minutes.

Note: this gives a small portion. This recipe won't work with fresh pineapple juice as it contains an enzyme that inactivates the gelatine.

KIDNEY AND CARROT

1 lambs kidney
a little sunflower oil
½ small carrot (peeled and cubed)
½ small stick celery (chopped)

½ potato (peeled and diced)
½ tsp yeast extract dissolved in 125ml (¼ pint) of water

Cut kidney in half and remove core. Heat oil in pan and brown kidney on all sides very quickly. Remove and cut into small pieces. Return to pan and add all other ingredients. Boil and then simmer 20–30 minutes.

LEEK BROTH

1 small leek (tough leaves removed, cleaned and thinly sliced)
100g (4oz) turnips or swede (peeled and diced)

Put ingredients in a small pan with just enough water to cover. Bring to the boil and simmer for 20 minutes. Drain, reserving cooking liquid. Mash, adding enough of the cooking liquid to give the consistency you want.

Note: you could substitute potato for the turnip or swede. Add half a sliced carrot to the ingredients.

BABY'S LIVER

100g (4oz) lambs liver
2 tsp sunflower oil
2 medium courgettes (thinly sliced)
4 medium carrots (thinly sliced)

Steam carrots for 25 minutes, and courgettes for 15 minutes. Meanwhile, brown liver in a pan with the oil. Simmer with a little water (or stock) for 5–10 minutes until tender. Blend all ingredients together.

Note: depending on your baby's appetite, this will make up to four portions. Remainders can be frozen in individual portions for future use.

MEAT LOAF

100g (4oz) finely minced steak
2 small carrots (peeled and finely chopped)
small slice of onion (finely chopped)
2 tbsp water

Mix meat and vegetables and put in small oiled casserole or loaf tin with the water. Cover mixture with sheet of foil and bake at 180°C, 350°F, gas 4, for 45–60 minutes.

MILLET PORRIDGE

1 cup millet (choose flaked grains)
3 cups liquid (use water, milk or milk and water)

Wash the millet by running fresh water through it in a sieve or colander. Add the millet to the liquid and heat to boiling. Lid the pan and simmer for about 20 minutes.

Note: this is quite chewy, and it has a pleasant, nutty flavour.

SUPER DE-LUXE MUESLI

750g (1½lbs) porridge oats
500g (1lb) wheat flakes
50g (2oz) coconut flakes
150g (6oz) dried apricots (chopped finely)
50g (2oz) pumpkin seeds (or sesame seeds)
50g (2oz) pine kernels (or sunflower seeds)
100g (4oz) sultanas

Mix all these ingredients together. Add milk to make the consistency preferred at the time of serving and leave to stand for five minutes. Mix again and add more milk if necessary. Babies may need the mixture blended.

Note: this makes a very large quantity for storing dry in a stone or glass jar. Try a peeled and cored dessert pear with a sprinkling of muesli, blended, as a change.

NECTARINE OR PEACH PUD

1 ripe peach or nectarine (skinned, halved and stoned)
1 tbsp natural yoghurt
½ banana (mashed)

Mash or sieve the fruit to the texture your baby prefers. Add to the banana and yoghurt.

NUT LOAF

50g (2oz) ground nuts (unsalted peanuts hazelnuts, almonds)
1 tbsp tomato purée
½ small onion (finely chopped)
½ egg (beaten)
50g (2oz) wholemeal breadcrumbs
pinch mixed spice

Cook onion in a small amount of water for 5 minutes. Drain and add tomato purée. Add egg, breadcrumbs, nuts and spice and stir well. Bake in an oiled casserole at 180°C, 350°F, gas 4, for 30 minutes.

Note: double quantities for 2 adults and a baby.

OATS AND PEAR

1 small pear (peeled and cored)
1 tbsp (rounded) fine oatmeal or rolled oats (put through the blender or grinder)
1–2 tbsp milk

Mix this and serve as it is. For younger babies just beginning on solid food, cook for 2 minutes, stirring constantly.

PANCAKES

570ml (1 pint) milk
2 eggs
200g (8oz) plain flour (wholemeal)
small amount sunflower oil

Mix the milk, eggs and flour thoroughly to make a runny batter. Oil a frying pan and add 2 tbsp of batter per pancake. Cook for 2 minutes, turn and cook on the other side for 2 minutes or slightly less. This quantity makes about 12 thin pancakes

Note: for filling ideas, choose between grated cheese, puréed apple, peas, mashed banana with a little yoghurt. Place filling in centre of pancake and roll up.

PASTA AND VEGETABLE SAUCE

150g (6oz) small pasta (eg shells, macaroni)
2 tbsp sunflower oil
1 medium onion (finely chopped)
½ green or red pepper (finely chopped)
50g (2oz) mushrooms (finely chopped)
50g (2oz) carrot (grated or finely chopped)
1 tbsp plain flour
275ml (½ pint) water, milk or milk and water

Cook pasta according to directions on packet. Heat oil and sweat onion, pepper, mushrooms and carrot, with pan lid on, for 10–15 minutes, until the vegetables are soft. Add flour, mix well, cook for one minute. Remove from heat and gradually add liquid. Boil to thicken, stirring all the time. Add pasta.

Note: this will serve 2 adults and a baby – the adults will want their portions seasoned. A crispy topping of 25g (1oz) finely grated cheese added to 25g (1oz) wholemeal breadcrumbs, browned under the grill, adds to the taste and nutritional value of this dish.

BABY'S PLUM PUDDING

4 ripe plums (peeled and stoned)
1 tbsp natural yoghurt
1 tsp desiccated coconut

Stew for about 5 minutes in a small amount of water and then mash or sieve. Add to yoghurt and coconut.

Note: choose ripe plums at the height of the season to avoid a bitter taste.

RICE, CHICKEN AND CABBAGE

1 chicken piece (skinned)
stick of celery (chopped)
parsley stalks

Place chicken in pan with water to cover. Add celery and parsley.

Simmer gently in lidded pan for 30 minutes. Drain and reserve liquid for cooking rice (see recipe). Bone chicken if necessary and chop. Serve mixed with rice and cabbage (see recipe).

BABY'S RISOTTO

50g (2oz) rice (cooked)
25g (1oz) carrots (chopped and cooked)
25g (1oz) peas (cooked)
small piece of chicken (cooked and chopped)

Mix all the ingredients together, and if a little dry, moisten with a small amount of natural yoghurt.

Note: cook the vegetables with the rice to save time. Carrots and rice start off together; add the peas halfway through the cooking time.

RUSKS

Cut up wholemeal bread into fingers – about 2cm (one inch) wide. Dry out in a slow oven (150°C, 300°F, gas 2) for 20 minutes to make a hard rusk that's still fairly moist on the inside. If you use thick bread, you may need extra time in the oven.

SESAME FINGERS

150g (6oz) wholemeal flour
50g (2oz) sesame seeds
½ cup sunflower oil
½ cup water

Mix ingredients to form a stiff dough. Roll out to 50mm (¼ inch) thickness and cut into finger shapes. Place on greased baking tray and bake at 180°C, 350°F, gas 4, for 15–20 minutes.

FAMILY WINTER SOUP

1 medium onion (finely chopped)
2 carrots (sliced)
1 parsnip (sliced)

1 small turnip (chopped)
2 medium potatoes (peeled and sliced)
2 sticks celery (chopped)
175g (7oz) tinned tomatoes
570ml (1 pint) water
bouquet garni
black pepper
small amount of sunflower oil

Sauté onion in oil for 3 minutes. Add remaining ingredients. Bring to boil. Simmer 30–45 minutes. Add salt to adult portions. Put in food processor or blend if preferred.

Note: substitute milk for some of the water for a richer soup.

SPREADS

Try these ideas:
• grated low-fat cheese (eg Edam) mashed with avocado
• mashed hard-boiled egg yolk with natural yoghurt
• cottage cheese and grated carrot
• grated cheese, finely grated carrot and yoghurt
• cooked and drained split red lentils mixed with tomato purée and cottage cheese (freezes well if you have too much for immediate use)

STEWED APPLE AND YOGHURT

1 dessert apple (peeled, cored and chopped)
1 tbsp natural yoghurt

Put the apple into a pan with a very small amount of water. Simmer for 5–10 minutes until tender. Mash. Stir in yoghurt.

Note: the same recipe can be used for pears, nectarines, peaches and apricots. You can bake the fruit instead – an economical way of using fuel if you have the oven already on for another dish. In a medium oven, place the whole, cored apple in an ovenproof dish, with a small amount of water, for about 20 minutes. Peel when cooked and then sieve or mash.

STOCK FOR BABIES

Meat bones (chicken, lamb, beef)
1 carrot
1 stick celery
bouquet garni

Cover bones and other ingredients with cold water. Bring to the boil and remove any fat from the top. Simmer with lid on for 3 hours, adding more liquid if the water gets too low. Use at once or store in fridge for 2–3 days, or freeze.

BABY'S SUMMER CUP

1 peach (peeled and stoned)
equal quantities of milk and pineapple juice, up to about ½ cup

Blend or food process until smooth.

PAT'S WHOLEMEAL BREAD

200g (8oz) wholemeal flour (plain)
½ tsp salt (level)
12½g (½oz) fresh yeast
125ml (¼ pint) tepid water (approximately)
25mg tablet ascorbic acid (this is vitamin C in tablet form – available from the chemist. Its use speeds up the rising process and improves the bread's texture)

Sieve flour and add salt. Dissolve ascorbic acid tablet in water. Blend the fresh yeast in water. Add liquid to flour and mix to a dough. Knead thoroughly on lightly floured surface. Heat oven to 230°C, 450°F, gas 8. Shape dough into small loaf or 6–8 buns. Put in a large polythene bag to rise, and tie loosely. Leave until doubles in size. Remove polythene bag and place loaf in tin or buns on tray. Bake loaf 30–35 minutes, buns 15–20 minutes.

Note: to make a larger quantity, double all ingredients except yeast and ascorbic acid. You may need more or less liquid – go by the 'feel' of your dough. It should become smooth and not sticky.

HOME-MADE YOGHURT

500g (18oz) whole milk
1 tbsp dried milk powder
1 tbsp natural yoghurt

Mix the milk with the powder and heat to boiling point. Leave to cool until hand-hot. Mix in the yoghurt and whisk well. Put the mixture into a wide-necked vacuum flask and leave for 6 hours. Pour contents into a clean airtight container and stir well. Lid the container or seal with Clingfilm. Refrigerate 4–6 hours before use. Keeps for about a week.

Note: reserve a little from each batch you make as the next batch's starter.

USEFUL ADDRESSES

NATIONAL CHILDBIRTH TRUST Alexandra House, Oldham Terrace, London W3 6NH. Telephone 01 992 8637. See local phone book for branches or contact headquarters.
In addition to antenatal classes and postnatal support groups, NCT has a network of breastfeeding counsellors who will give support and information to any mother with a query about breastfeeding. Leaflets available.
THE ASSOCIATION OF BREASTFEEDING MOTHERS 131 Mayow Road, London SE26 4HZ. Telephone 01 778 4769 for a recorded list of ABM counsellors in the UK.
Breastfeeding support, counselling and leaflets. Local ABM groups hold regular meetings.
LA LECHE LEAGUE GREAT BRITAIN BM 3424, London WC1N 3XX. Telephone 01 242 1278.
LLL is an international organisation with branches in many countries. LLL leaders run local groups and give breastfeeding information and support. Newsletter and leaflets.
DISABLED LIVING FOUNDATION 380–384 Harrow Road, London W9 2HU. Telephone 01 289 6111.
Information on the practicalities of living with a disability, including information for parents of handicapped babies with feeding problems.
THE VEGAN SOCIETY 33–35 George Street, Oxford OX1 2AY. Telephone 0865 722166.
Leaflets and advice on diets that exclude all animal products.
THE VEGETARIAN SOCIETY Parkdale, Durham Road, Altrincham, Cheshire WA14 4QG. Telephone 061 928 0793.
Information and advice on vegetarian diets and cooking.
CLEFT LIP AND PALATE ASSOCIATION (CLAPA) 1 Eastwood Gardens, Kenton, Newcastle-upon-Tyne NE3 3DQ. Telephone 0632 859396.
Counselling and support for parents of newborn babies with cleft lips or palates.

COELIAC SOCIETY OF THE UNITED KINGDOM PO Box 220, High Wycombe, Buckinghamshire HP11 2HY. Telephone 0494 37278.
Information and advice through a network of about 70 groups.
FOUNDATION FOR THE STUDY OF INFANT DEATH (Cot Death Research and Support Associations) 15 Belgrave Street, London SW1X 8PS. Telephone 01 235 1712.
Advice and counselling for newly bereaved parents. Sponsors research and produces useful leaflets.
BMAC (BABY MILK ACTION COALITION) 34 Blinco Grove, Cambridge CB1 4TS. Telephone 0223 210094.

NURSING MOTHERS ASSOCIATION OF AUSTRALIA PO Box 231, Nunawading, Victoria 3131, Australia.
LA LECHE LEAGUE IN AUSTRALIA c/o Finky McKay, 8 Gateshead Drive, Wantirna, Victoria 3152, Australia.
KARITANE MOTHERCRAFT SOCIETY 171 Avoca Street, Randwick, NSW 2031, Australia.
Help for mothers with problem babies either through their clinic or hospital.

PLUNKET SOCIETY 3 Moncrief Street, Mount Victoria, Wellington, New Zealand. Telephone 04 844 973
A nationwide network of centres providing advice and assistance for all aspects of childbirth.
LA LECHE LEAGUE IN NEW ZEALAND Box 13 383, Wellington 4, New Zealand. Telephone 04 785 213.
Information and support for women wishing to breastfeed their babies.
WELLINGTON HYPER-ACTIVITY AND ALLERGY ASSOCIATION 93 Waipapa Road, Wellington, New Zealand. Telephone 04 862 514.
Information and advice on hyper-activity and allergy problems among babies and children.

BOOKLIST

There are many books available on breastfeeding, and on feeding and caring for a baby and/or the family. A selection of the ones I would recommend, and which have formed the background for this book are:

Carr, Janet, *Helping Your Handicapped Child* (London: Penguin 1980)

Graham, Louise, *A Good Start – Healthy Eating in the First Five Years* (London: Penguin 1986)

Hanssen, M., *E for Additives* (Thorsons 1987)

Helsing, E and Savage-King, F., *Breastfeeding in Practice* (London: OUP 1982)

Holt, Kenneth S. and Brant, H. A., *The Complete Mothercare Manual* (London: Conran Octopus 1986)

Hull, Sylvia, *Cooking for a Baby* (London: Penguin 1979)

Jolly, Hugh, *The Book of Child Care* (London: Unwin Hyman 1975)

Kinman, Jenny, *Going on to Solids* (London: Paperfronts 1987)

Lewis, Catherine, *Growing up with Good Food* (London: Unwin Hyman 1982)

Messenger, Máire, *The Breastfeeding Book* (London: Century 1982)

Minchin, Maureen, *Breastfeeding Matters* (London: Alma Publications 1985)

Minchin, Maureen, *Food for Thought – a parents' guide to food intolerance* (London: OUP 1986)

Stanway, Andrew and Stanway, Penny, *Breast is Best* (London: Pan 1978)

Templeton, Louise, *The Right Food for your Kids* (London: Century 1984)

The research reports which include the breastfeeding rates to be found on page 22 are from:

Jones, D. A., *Social Science and Medicine* (1986) pages 11, 26, 1151–1156

Jones, D. A., *Midwifery* (1986) pages 2, 141–146

London Food Commission. *Warding Off the Bottle* (1986)

ACTIVE BIRTH

Janet Balaskas

Janet Balaskas is a childbirth educator, author and activist, and is the founder of the International Active Birth Movement. She trained with the National Childbirth Trust and organised the Birthrights Rally and two International Conferences on Active Birth in London in 1982/3. She has campaigned for women to have the right to choose an active birth and has helped to effect change in maternity practices and midwifery education internationally.

This practical, compassionate and informative handbook, which includes birth accounts of many women, will help you prepare for an active childbirth.

NEW MOTHERS AT WORK

Julia Brannen and Peter Moss

You have just had your baby and have decided to go back to work. You question yourself about your decision; you don't know what will be for the best – for your baby, your family and for you. Now you have to plan for childcare, and you are worried and anxious about the problems that may arise at work.

The working mother in Britain today has to run an obstacle course of decision-making and organisation. NEW MOTHERS AT WORK presents a true picture of the emotional and practical problems that face her. It

- discusses the financial and career factors which influence decisions on work and childcare
- explores emotional factors including common feelings of guilt
- offers a wealth of practical strategies from the first-hand accounts of others
- provides an invaluable source of material for those in the fields of women's studies, employment and childcare

The authors, Julia Brannen and Peter Moss, are both parents themselves and have worked for many years at the Thomas Coram Research Unit, Institute of Education, University of London.

THE ILLUSTRATED DICTIONARY OF PREGNANCY AND BIRTH

Heather Welford

The Illustrated Dictionary of Pregnancy and Birth has over 450 entries – from Alphafetoprotein to Old Wives' Tales; Apgar Test to Maternity Leave; Braxton-Hicks Contractions to Zygote; Dental Checks to Vernix – and many clear and helpful illustrations. Comprehensive and straightforward, it includes everything you'll need to know for a happy, healthy pregnancy and birth.

Heather Welford is a mother, and freelance journalist specialising in the areas of pregnancy, health and child care. She writes regularly for Parents magazine. She has called on experience and research, and the advice of a leading obstetrician and a midwife to compile all the information both a new or experienced mother could want, in an attractive and accessible format.

BOOK OF CHILD CARE
The complete guide for today's parents

Hugh Jolly

'...the only babycare book on the market to tell you all you need to know about the care and development of your child in one volume.'

Parents magazine

'...as comprehensive a guide as any parent could wish for.'
Mother magazine

'Dr Jolly is first-class on lumps and bumps and spots and rashes. He is superb on accidents and illnesses, and authoritative on children in hospital.'
Times Educational Supplement

'...the most comprehensive guide to all aspects of looking after children.'
Daily Mail

'The best of the many books on the subject are those which emphasise that babies are individual human beings ... as does Dr Hugh Jolly in the latest edition of his **Book of Child Care**.'
The Lancet

YOUR LIFE AFTER BIRTH

Exercises and Meditations for the First Year of Motherhood

Paddy O'Brien

This positive and practical handbook draws on women's own accounts of their post-natal feelings and experiences, and provides a comprehensive programme of relaxation, guided fantasy, assertiveness and self-defence to help you grow stronger emotionally as well as physically.

It provides practical, mental and physical exercises to help you cope with tiredness and the new demands on your time and emotions, and to make positive plans for *yourself* as well as the baby. It helps you to rediscover your own needs and desires, to express your feelings about the experience of having a child and what this does to your body, and to make realistic decisions about whether to have another child. It also includes women's moving accounts of their experiences of stillbirth and one mother's feelings about the challenge of caring for her handicapped child.

A sequel to BIRTH AND OUR BODIES, this essential post-natal companion guide is based on the author's successful classes and is organised for you to use alone, in pairs or in groups.

BIRTH AND OUR BODIES

Exercises and Meditations for the Childbearing Year and Preparation for Active Birth

Paddy O'Brien

This practical and positive companion guide provides women with detailed physical and mental exercises to practise through pregnancy and birth

Working chronologically from the time when a woman may not even be pregnant but hopes to conceive in the near future, right through to the birth itself, the guide provides a comprehensive exercise programme for relaxation, combating morning sickness, stage fright in the last few weeks of pregnancy and for strengthening the pelvic floor muscles.

Illustrated with line drawings taken from 'life' both in the exercise classes which Paddy O'Brien runs, and at the time of the birth itself, BIRTH AND OUR BODIES helps mothers to stay in touch with a body, and in charge of it, when it seems in danger of being taken over by the baby. So, as well as maintaining and strengthening your muscles you get stronger and more supple emotionally.

This is a pocket-sized companion, easy to use at home, or at work – it encourages the participation of partners and can be used too whenever you have time to yourself.

'a gem, beautifully presented and designed, clear without being patronising.'

Helen Roberts

YOUR BODY, YOUR BABY, YOUR LIFE

Angela Phillips
with Nicky Lean and Barbara Jacobs

Your Body, Your Baby, Your Life starts with help on planning for pregnancy six months before you conceive, stays with you up to and through the birth and sees you safely into the world of new parenthood. It equips you with the information you need to work *with* health professionals, giving you a voice in your own care and allowing you to make decisions about the pregnancy and labour *you* want. It includes information on:

- choices in ante-natal treatment and the place of birth
- preparing yourself mentally and physically for childbirth
- recognising problems and assessing the help you are offered
- tests and their side effects
- understanding your rights and claiming benefits
- your body after pregnancy
- living with a new baby
- returning to work and much more!

'At last a book for the mother which regards her as a real person'

Anna Raeburn

'answers all those questions \ .. you'd only dare ask your best friend. The horrors of feeling like a stranded whale, going off sex and wanting to cry all the time are all taken in the book's stride and Ros Asquith's cartoons don't let you forget the funny side of it all ... it makes having a baby sound like fun, not an illness'

Company

'this baby book could be your best friend'

Mother magazine

'A landmark in its field'

Jean Shapiro of *Good Housekeeping*

'Among the best pregnancy books we've ever seen'

Parents magazine

Also by Unwin Paperbacks and Pandora Press

Book of Child Care   *Hugh Jolly* .... £8.95☐
Illustrated Dictionary of Pregnancy and Birth
Heather Welford .... £3.95☐
Sleep Well   *Marc Weissbluth* .... £3.95☐
Understanding Children's Problems   *Penny Jacques* .... £3.50☐
Birth Matters: Issues and alternatives in Childbirth
Roz Claxton (Ed) .... £3.95☐
Active Birth   *Janet Balaskas* .... £3.95☐
New Mothers at Work   *Peter Moss & Julia Brannen* .... £5.95☐
Your Life After Birth: Exercises and meditations for the
    first year of motherhood   *Paddy O'Brien* .... £4.95☐
Birth and Our Bodies   *Paddy O'Brien* .... £3.95☐
Your Body, Your Baby, Your Life
Angela Phillips with Nicky Lean and Barbara Jacobs .... £4.50☐

All these books are available at your local bookshop or newsagent, or can be ordered direct by post. Just tick the titles you want and fill in the form below.

Name ....

Address ....

....

....

Write to Unwin Cash Sales, PO Box 11, Falmouth, Cornwall TR10 9EN.

Please enclose remittance to the value of the cover price plus:

UK: 60p for the first book plus 25p for the second book, thereafter, 15p for each additional book ordered to a maximum charge of £1.90.

BFPO and EIRE: 60p for the first book plus 25p for the second book and 15p for the next 7 books and thereafter 9p per book.

OVERSEAS INCLUDING EIRE: £1.25 for the first book plus 75p for the second book and 28p for each additional book.

Unwin Paperbacks reserve the right to show new retail prices on covers which may differ from those previously advertised in the text or elsewhere. Postage rates are also subject to revision.